Doing Disability Research in Africa

Gubela Mji
Editor

Doing Disability Research in Africa

Reflections from the African Network for Evidence-to-Action in Disability (AfriNEAD)

palgrave
macmillan

Editor
Gubela Mji
Cape Town, South Africa

ISBN 978-3-031-98548-5 ISBN 978-3-031-98549-2 (eBook)
https://doi.org/10.1007/978-3-031-98549-2

This Palgrave Macmillan imprint is published by the registered company Springer Nature Switzerland AG
The registered company address is: Gewerbestrasse 11, 6330 Cham, Switzerland

I dedicate this book to those whose knowledge and world view cannot be integrated into the mainstream of knowledge systems because of their marginalization.

Foreword

The African Network for Evidence-to-Action in Disability (AfriNEAD) is one of the instruments which deserve acknowledgement in making a priceless contribution, in the equalization of opportunities for persons with disabilities. We would be the first to agree, however, that this journey started long before, with the Standard Rules on the Equalization of Opportunities for Persons with Disabilities (December 20, 1993), Protocol to the African Charter on Human and Rights of Women in Africa July 11, 2002, and the UN Convention on the Rights of Persons with Disabilities (CRPD, December 13, 2006).

Despite a slow and often faltering evolution, the situation of persons with disabilities worldwide is now starting to make small and incremental positive changes. We are in a new and exciting era of awareness, activity, transformation and commitment in the sphere of disability, both in Africa, and beyond.

Now there is a need for focus in specific regions, persons with disabilities in Africa championed and led by Disability Movement are not yet experiencing meaningful change in their quality of life, access to equal rights, economic opportunities and level of community integration, despite a favourable policy environment in some countries and a supportive research evidence base.

Research evidence alone cannot achieve the task of ensuring that evidence is translated, particularly in the pan-African context, to ensure that it makes an impact at policy level to assist and improve conditions at grassroots level for the realization of rights of persons with disabilities in the region. To address this, AfriNEAD brought to the table a wide range of stakeholders that can assist in the process of research in specific areas, ranging from asking the appropriate research questions through to utilizing the research outcomes. Recognizing the important role of research and researchers, the time is now to develop the capacity of researchers with disabilities. Central to capacitating researchers with disabilities with research skills is the slogan, "Nothing About Us Without Us" by Krzysztof Kieslowski, 1972, 'the intention of the slogan is to ensure that persons with disabilities supported by their Movement lead the experiences that are about their lives'.

AfriNEAD has developed a platform with different roles that can be played by persons with disabilities. This paradigm requires capacitating persons with disabilities with research skills that will assist them to take their rightful position of sometimes acting as leaders of disability research. There is a generation of young people with disabilities who are preparing themselves to play this role. AfriNEAD has presented a possibility of a dream of an equitable future where ALL can play interchangeable roles. This book presents the testimony of this possibility.

I congratulate the editor and authors of this landmark volume for the excellent and important work. May AfriNEAD be a learning lesson and a springboard for other similar disability research networks to help propel this kind of development in the region.

Cape Town, South Africa
October 2024

Mzolisi Toni

Declaration

By submitting this draft book electronically, I declare that the entirety of the work contained therein is my own, original work and that of the authors that supported me to write some of the chapters. Authors that have contributed to the chapters have been mentioned. Publications cited in the book have been included in the reference list. I have not previously in its entirety submitted this book to any other publisher except for Palgrave.

October 2024 Gubela Mji

Acknowledgements

This book is about a collective thought regarding how a network could be used as a prong for the realization of rights for persons with disabilities in Africa and as such there is need to acknowledge these various people that contributed to the development of the network. As disability researchers and practitioners, we have been inspired by a range of people especially disabled people's organizations from the region who created a springboard and assisted in providing leadership for the development of AfriNEAD and the writing of this book. These disability activists and scholars have in recent years guided the network to remain focused on its twists and turns. They not only guided the network but also shaped our thinking about disability, challenging us to imagine an inclusive future that give human dignity and respect to ALL.

The early stages of the development of AfriNEAD would have been difficult without the guidance of people from the Disability Rights Movement: Chairpersons of Southern Africa Federation of the Disabled SAFOD: Mr Alexander Phiri, Dr Rachel Kachaje and Mr Mussa Chiwaula. They were Chairpersons of SAFOD at various times and all three are deceased—may their souls rest in peace. Others are Mr Mzolisi Toni who was the Chairperson of DPSA, played a critical role in linking AfriNEAD organizers with critical disability stakeholders; Mr AK Dube the Chairperson of the then African Decade for persons with disabilities, now known as African Disability Alliance (ADA); Mr Shuaib Chalklen, the Chairperson of African Disability Forum (ADF) and The Western

Cape Network for persons with Disability, in particular: Mr Rustim Ariefdien, Mr Anthony Ghillino, Dr Michelle Botha, Mr Vincent Daniels and Ms Hillary Lane. These colleagues are commended for the support and energy they gave the network to ensure its success.

We also received support from our regional Colleagues, and I would like to mention Prof Anthony Edusei from Kwame Nkrumah University of Science and Technology in Kumasi, Ghana and Prof Tsitsi Chataika from University of Zimbabwe, Zimbabwe.

Our international partners have given a push to the development of AfriNEAD and hence the writing of this book. Prof Mac MacLachlan from Trinity College Dublin School of Psychology and Centre for Global Health, Dublin, Ireland, now based at the Maynooth University, Maynooth, CO. Kildare, Ireland, Prof Arne Eide SINTEF, in Oslo Norway, Prof Nora Groce, University College of London, London, UK, Prof Patrick Devlieger Ku Leuven University, Leuven, Belgium and Prof Mark Harniss Washington University, Seattle, Washington, United States. All these international partners contributed their time and expertise to allow the network to grow. The Disability Studies Unit at the University of Cape Town, Cape Town, South Africa, and different units and departments at Stellenbosch University, Stellenbosch, South Africa, had played a critical role in assisting AfriNEAD to grow. We owe a great deal to the Disability Unit, Department of Psychology and the Division of Disability and Rehabilitation Studies for their support for AfriNEAD and the writing of this book.

I would like to acknowledge Clelia Petracca the Commissioning Editor—Disability Studies for Palgrave for her support and encouragement in authoring this book. Lastly, I want to thank my family for their patience in writing this book.

Cape Town, South Africa
October 2024

Gubela Mji

About this Book

The aim of this book is to present a history of the African Network for Evidence-to-Action in Disability (AfriNEAD) on its quest to be a regional network. AfriNEAD is a regional disability research network founded in 2007 and based at the Division of Disability and Rehabilitation Studies (DDRS) in the Medicine and Health Science Faculty, Stellenbosch University, Stellenbosch, South Africa. AfriNEAD's mission is to facilitate the dynamic exchange of ideas about disability research evidence to advance the realization of equal rights of persons with disabilities and promote action for social inclusion and participation. AfriNEAD's vision is that it will become a significant contributor and facilitator regarding the needs of persons with disabilities in Africa, by assisting in translating existing and new research in the disability arena into meaningful evidence-based advocacy, practice, products and policy.

AfriNEAD is one of networks in Africa that works toward breaking down operation silos among various stakeholders involved in addressing issues affecting persons with disabilities. It has also developed several strategic partnerships at national and regional levels within Africa, as well as with partners further abroad. Being based at the DDRS with its focus on postgraduate disability and rehabilitation programs, AfriNEAD draws postgraduate students with disabilities from across Africa for the advancement of disability and rehabilitation studies within the African region and beyond. Further, it brings to this network experienced disability researchers to develop regional, multi-country disability research projects that influence policy and practice for the realization of the rights of persons with disabilities in Africa.

AfriNEAD is an inclusive grassroots network that has managed to put central to its intention persons with disabilities and debunked the perception that research is something elusive that is only discussed by a few. The network is aware of the work that has been done by persons with disabilities in the realization of their rights and some of their contributions made in global organizations such as the UN on the development of human rights documents, such as the Convention on the Rights of Persons with Disabilities (CRPD) of 2006. It further affirms the strength of persons with disabilities by drawing on their skills in the co-creation of AfriNEAD.

To facilitate a disability network in Africa is not an easy journey due to infra-structure and internet connectivity challenges. For example, some persons with disabilities in most African countries do not have safety nets such as social security. Persons with disabilities bear the extra burden of being unable to compete equally in the open labour market. These issues are exacerbated by intersecting problems related to poor governance and poverty. Despite these challenges AfriNEAD persisted, the proposed book will chart the path that AfriNEAD leadership took to develop the network, the guiding principles, the accomplishments achieved through its efforts and a pathway to the future.

Much as there has been rapid growth and development in networking and globalization, minimal information exists about the conceptualization and sustainability of networks, especially within the African region. A text that integrates a history of AfriNEAD with lessons learnt would be very useful to young researchers, giving them information on how to initiate and sustain an inclusive disability network. The book will also not only recount the story of AfriNEAD but also give a critical analysis of the growth of a disability research initiative.

The sustainability of this disability network is linked to drawing strength from African principles and concepts. These concepts and principles have been interwoven to create a resilient spiderweb that could sustain the network through difficult times.

Cape Town, South Africa
October 2024

Gubela Mji

Contents

Editor and Contributors

About the Editor

Gubela Mji holds a PhD in Family Medicine from Stellenbosch University, Stellenbosch, South Africa. She is an emeritus professor and a previous director for the Division of Disability and Rehabilitation Studies (DDRS) at Stellenbosch University, Stellenbosch, South Africa. Originally a physiotherapist by profession, she has translated this into disability and rehabilitation studies. An NRF-rated researcher, her work focuses on disability, indigenous knowledge systems and rural health.

On June 29, 2015, she produced a Ted talk on Table Mountain on how we can make disability research accessible in Africa. She recently edited the book: The walk without limbs searching for indigenous health knowledge in rural South Africa which can be accessed from https://books.aosis.co.za/index.php/ob/catalog/book/. She advanced the academic scholarship of Stellenbosch University, Stellenbosch, South Africa, by supporting the DDRS to become a regional hub for interdisciplinary debates on disability, rehabilitation and indigenous knowledge systems, offering postgraduate diplomas, master's and PhD studies. Increasingly, a diversified student population has emerged within this field contributing significantly to the university's strategic aim of engaged scholarship through community interaction.

It is within this quest for local, regional and international understanding of disability and poverty that she supported the development of the African Network for Evidence-to-Action in Disability (AfriNEAD) (www.sun.ac.za/AfriNEAD) in 2007 at Stellenbosch University, Stellenbosch, South Africa. She was the Chairperson of AfriNEAD until the end of the year 2023. The focus of AfriNEAD is the translation of disability research into action for direct impact on policy and practice, thus impacting on the lives of persons with disabilities. The network had been in existence for 17 years in 2023 and hosts the African Journal of Disability (www.ajod.org).

In her retirement, she intends to continue with her quest of being a global scholar beyond her formal employment at Stellenbosch University, Stellenbosch, South Africa. She wants to focus on research that decolonizes indigenous knowledge systems and disability studies with the goal of emancipating and decolonizing these knowledge systems in Africa.

Contributors

Rosemary Choma holds a master's degree in project management and is pursuing a PhD in health and Rehabilitation Sciences at Stellenbosch University, Stellenbosch, South Africa. She transitioned into a college tutor and secretarial expert before serving in various local and international roles. As founder of ADOT (https://www.adot.or.tz), she advocates for disability rights and coordinates Tanzanead (https://www/tanzanead.org). She represented Tanzania at the 7th AfriNEAD Conference in 2023. She also is the author of *This Is Me.*

Patrick Devlieger is a retired professor from KU Leuven University, Leuven, Belgium. His academic background is in education and anthropology. His research field started in the DR Congo, followed by research in Zimbabwe, United States, and South Africa. He held associate positions at the University of Illinois, Urbana-Champaign, United States, University of Alberta, Edmonton, Canada and Stellenbosch University, Stellenbosch, South Africa. He had written on the linguistic, social-historical, and material contexts of people with disabilities. He also conducted research on the material conditions of people with leprosy in several countries.

Nomvo Dwadwa-Henda holds a PhD in Health Sciences Rehabilitation and is a post-doctoral fellow at the Division of Disability and Rehabilitation Studies, Stellenbosch University, Stellenbosch, South Africa. Her research interests are in disability inclusion, indigenous knowledge and health, gender-based violence.

Anthony Edusei a professor, holds a PhD in Human Nutrition, MSc. in Applied Human Nutrition and a Master of Public Health Degree. He is an emeritus professor with 27 years of experience in teaching and research in Health Promotion and Disability Studies in the School of Public Health and Medicine and Dentistry in Kwame Nkrumah University of Science and Technology, Kumasi, Ghana.

Callista Kahonde has a background in Physiotherapy and a PhD in Disability Studies. She is a senior lecturer in the Division of Disability and Rehabilitation Studies at Stellenbosch University, Stellenbosch in South Africa. Her research interests include intellectual and developmental disabilities within the context of the family, inclusive research methods and sexuality and reproductive education.

Hillary Lane was the previous coordinator of AfriNEAD. She is now retired. Her life has been about supporting other people with different degrees of disabilities, to reach their full potential as active members of society. She is now the chairperson of South African Riding (horse riding) for the Disabled and takes great pleasure in being part of shaping the lives of the next generation.

Victor Locoro was a lecturer of special needs education and community-based rehabilitation at Kyambogo University, Kampala, Uganda for many years. His area of work focus is education and rehabilitation of children with complex communication needs arising from multisensory impairments. He is now a consultant in disability inclusive education and development work.

Marcia Lyner-Cleophas holds a PhD in Psychology from Stellenbosch University, Stellenbosch, South Africa. She is the head of Disability Unit, Stellenbosch University, Stellenbosch, South Africa, and member of AfriNEAD, SAACDHE, HEDSA and a Change Ability Management Committee. As an educational psychologist, she is registered with the HPCSA, has written a few peer-reviewed journal articles and chapters as well as reviewed masters and doctoral theses in the disability body of work.

Malcolm MacLachlan is a professor of Psychology and Social inclusion and co-director of all the ALL (Assisting Living & Learning) Institute at Maynooth University, Ireland. He was also the clinical lead for the

National Clinical program for People with disabilities in the Irish Health Services.

Nondwe Mlenzana holds a PhD (Physiotherapy) and is an associate professor at the Department of Physiotherapy, University of the Western Cape, Cape Town, South Africa. She is a member of AfriNEAD and the Disability Research Country working Groups (DRCWGs).

Alister Munthali a professor, holds an MA in Medical Anthropology from the University of Amsterdam, Amsterdam, Netherlands and a PhD in Anthropology from Rhodes University, Makhanda, South Africa. He works for PALM Consulting Limited. Previously, he worked for the University of Malawi, Zomba, Malawi, for more than 25 years. He has done research on disability since 2002.

Chioma Ohajunwa holds a PhD in Health Sciences Rehabilitation and is a senior lecturer at Africa Centre for HIV/AIDS Management, Faculty of Economic and Management Sciences, Stellenbosch University, Stellenbosch, South Africa. Her research interests are in disability, spirituality and inclusive health, indigenous knowledge, decoloniality/post-coloniality. She has published locally and internationally.

Washiela Sait holds a master's degree in Disability Studies from the University of Cape Town, Cape Town, South Africa, and PhD in Health Science Rehabilitation from Stellenbosch University, Stellenbosch, South Africa. Her youngest son's diagnosis of Duchenne Muscular Dystrophy in the 1980s truly ignited her passion for disability activism. She is currently volunteering at Disabled Children Action Group (DICAG) Western Cape, South Africa, to improve its organizational development.

Mzolisi Toni holds a master's degree in Disability Studies (University of Cape Town, Cape Town, South Africa) and an Honorary Doctorate for as a recognition of his efforts to advance disability rights in South Africa since early 1990s. He has contributed to the research in Xhosa & WHO International Classification of functioning, Disability and Health

Dagnachew Wakene is a Disability Rights consultant and lawyer, based in Ethiopia, holds MPhil (Stellenbosch University, Stellenbosch in South Africa), LLB (Addis Ababa University, Addis Ababa, Ethiopia), and is LLD candidate (University of Pretoria, Pretoria, South Africa). Latest publication: Marcia Rioux, Paula Pinto, Dagnachew Wakene, et al. Reinventing Activism: Evidence-based Participatory Monitoring as a Tool for Social Change. The Routledge Handbook of Disability Activism. Routledge (2020).

List of Figures

List of Tables

CHAPTER 1

The Quest to Develop an African Disability Research Network

Gubela Mji

1.1 Introduction

Persons with disabilities in Africa are not yet experiencing meaningful change in their quality of life, access to equal rights and level of community integration, despite a favourable policy environment in some countries and a supportive research evidence base (Kachaje et al., 2014). Real change and social development are still required to realize a truly inclusive society (Mji et al., 2009a, b). Inclusive policies that facilitate access to equal human rights will assist in unlocking the potential of persons with disabilities to make contributions to the development agenda in their various countries (MacLachlan et al., 2014).

Despite a slow and often faltering evolution, the situation of people with disabilities is now starting to be featured on the international development agenda (Mji et al., 2009a, b). We are in a new and exciting era of awareness, activity and commitment in the sphere of disability, both in Africa and beyond (Swartz, 2014). Many initiatives have placed disability

G. Mji (✉)
Cape Town, South Africa
e-mail: gumji@sun.ac.za

G. Mji (ed.), *Doing Disability Research in Africa*,
https://doi.org/10.1007/978-3-031-98549-2_1

as a matter of clear concern (Howel et al., 2006; Ingstad & White, 2007). Instruments such as United Nations Convention on the rights of Persons with disabilities (CRPD) and the Sustainable Development Goals (SDGs) with its 2030 agenda bring an excellent opportunity to work together towards the implementation of a common disability inclusion agenda and to accelerate the implementation of the CRPD (Panda, 2024; UN, 2006). These all hold the promise of contributing fundamental building blocks to realizing the rights of persons with disabilities in Africa (Kachaje et al., 2014). These lofty and worthy initiatives will be influenced by many factors. Their chances of success will be strengthened if they are powered by an evidence base that reaches into policy decisions and practical actions; which engages with persons with disabilities; through them, being with them and not only about them; and, where possible, being undertaken by them (Charlton, 1998; MacLachlan et al., 2014).

Various definitions of disability emphasize how it is society's lack of responsiveness to the needs of people with impairments that constitutes their disability rather than the nature of their impairment per se (Barnes & Mercer, 1997; Tilley et al., 2021). There is increasing evidence generated by research on disability that has been able to highlight factors that may facilitate the participation and inclusion of persons with disabilities in mainstream society (Balton et al., 2021). There is, however, a danger that the research community may simply accumulate evidence rather than translating this evidence to address the ways in which society can become more responsive to, and more inclusive of, persons with disabilities (Mji et al., 2009a, b). Such oversight would replicate the very circumstances that constitute the disabling environments that we aim to address. The challenge of translating research into evidence-based advocacy, practice and policy—particularly in the pan-African context—needs to be systematically addressed in a coherent and ongoing fashion (AfriNEAD Conferences, 2007, 2009, 2011, 2014, 2017, 2020, 2023).

In 2007, the Division of Disability and Rehabilitation Studies (DDRS) at Stellenbosch University (SU), Stellenbosch, South Africa, envisaged becoming a leading pan-African facilitator of evidence-to-action in disability by developing a regional disability research network (Mji et al., 2009a, b). Many networks exist and perform many different functions. For a network to be clearly beneficial to its members, those members need to be aware of the aims of the network and to understand that it uses a specific approach for a specific purpose (Dragon et al., 2008;

Friedman et al., 2007). The proposed network aimed to have representatives from as many African countries as possible and within each country it aimed to have representatives from as broad a range of stakeholders as possible, including PWDs, policymakers, practitioners and researchers (Kachaje et al., 2014; Mji et al., 2009a, b). Capitalizing then on the combined impetus afforded by the *African Decade for Disabled People* and the *United Nations Convention on the Rights of persons with disabilities*, the focus of the network was to be on how to combine research, policy and practice to realize the rights of persons with disabilities in the region. The African Network for Evidence-to-Action in disability (AfriNEAD) intended to respond to some of these concerns. The following section will address the rationale for the development of AfriNEAD.

1.2 Rationale for the Development of AfriNEAD

Despite the many progressive statements promulgated in recent years the extent of meaningful change in the actual quality of life of persons with disabilities in Africa remains limited. Even in a country with relative wealth, such as South Africa, where AfriNEAD was initiated. Despite the internationally acclaimed inclusive South African Constitution and established national strategies and policies (for instance from the South African Integrated National Disability Strategy White Paper, (1997); and the South African Employment Equity Act, 1998), the possibilities for persons with disabilities to have 'equal rights and dignity' remain distressingly illusive. In Africa, most persons with disabilities are not yet experiencing meaningful change in their quality of life, access to equal rights and level of community integration, despite a favourable policy environment and a limited, but supportive, research evidence base. Thus, the historical exclusion of persons with disabilities from society persists. Real change and social development are still required to realize a truly inclusive society (Mji et al., 2009a, b).

Translating research into evidence-based advocacy, policy, practice and products—particularly in the pan-African context—needed to be systematically addressed in a coordinated, coherent and consistent fashion. A wide range of stakeholders needed to be included in the process ranging from asking the appropriate research questions through to utilizing the research outcomes—that ultimately feed back into asking further relevant research questions. The UN Convention on the Rights of Persons with Disabilities (2006), which has now entered international law, was perhaps the most significant—moral and practical—step towards realizing the rights of persons with disabilities.

The Convention seeks to address discrimination, change perceptions and combat stereotypes and prejudices. Article 32 of the Convention states that 'Countries are to provide development assistance in efforts by developing countries to put into practice the Convention'. This article places an obligation on people in high-income countries to not only put the Convention into practice in their own countries but also to ensure that their countries also assist in putting it into action in low-income countries (AfriNEAD Conference, 2007, 2009, 2011, 2014, 2017, 2020, 2023).

The AfriNEAD initiative started by the DDRS at Stellenbosch University has been supported by its African civil society partner, the Secretariat of the African Decade for Persons with Disabilities, and its northern research partner, the Centre for Global Health, at Trinity College, Dublin, Ireland (Mji et al., 2009a, b). AfriNEAD has become a network with multiple partners and collaborators and seeks to become a significant contributor to addressing the needs of persons with disabilities in Africa (Kachaje et al., 2014). It seeks to achieve these needs by assisting in translating existing as well as new research in the disability arena into meaningful evidence-based advocacy, practice and products which can inform policy.

AfriNEAD, uniquely African in nature with intention of seeking solutions to its own obstacles and barriers within an African context, AfriNEAD can contribute to increasing the participation and inclusion of persons with disabilities in all aspects of society. AfriNEAD has done this by focusing on bridging the 'know-how' gap across a broad range of issues relevant to realizing the rights of persons with disabilities in Africa. AfriNEAD facilitates a multidimensional, intersectoral, interactive forum that focuses on how the evidence that is generated by disability researchers is translated to action (Mji et al., 2011). AfriNEAD also affords disability researchers exposure to the complexities of the issues of equity within the disability field and the need to see disability as a social and developmental issue.

AfriNEAD is a forum that builds and sustains relationships, partnerships and cooperation between researchers and users of research evidence and knowledge. The forum provides a platform where research results are better able to target and influence policy and practice. AfriNEAD lives in the research-policy-practice 'gaps' seen as 'problems' in other fora. Realizing that such 'problems' present the greatest opportunities for learning and enacting learning is the driving force behind AfriNEAD. It is within this regard that we introduce the African Network for Evidence-to-Action in Disability (AfriNEAD) and argue for its timeliness.

1.3 Process of Development of AfriNEAD Since Inauguration in 2007

AfriNEAD was developed at the Division of Disability and Rehabilitation Studies (DDRS) at Stellenbosch University, Stellenbosch, South Africa. The vision for AfriNEAD was that it will become a significant contributor to and facilitator around the needs of persons with disabilities in Africa, by assisting in translating existing and new research in the disability arena into meaningful evidence-based advocacy, practice, products and policy. The goal was to conduct research inclusively with the hope that this will breakdown the silos and hasten the realization of rights of PWDs within the region (Strnadová et al., 2022). Capitalizing on the combined impetus afforded by the CRPD (2006) and the African Decade for Persons with Disabilities in 1999, the focus of this network was on how to combine research, policy and practice to realize the rights of persons with disabilities in Africa (Kachaje et al., 2014; Mji et al., 2009a, b). To achieve this goal AfriNEAD developed six objectives to guide the network, and these are presented below:

1.3.1 Develop a Network to Facilitate and Coordinate Research Dialogue from Evidence-to-Action

AfriNEAD provides space for dialogue on critical disability issues, which has been facilitated by establishing a network whose primary objective was to explore effective ways of utilizing knowledge as a basis for planning action. The dialogue takes place between disabled people organisations (DPOs), academics, activists, practitioners, employers and civil servants from different parts of the African continent—all focused on the need to effect positive change in the quality of lives of persons with disabilities (Mji et al., 2009a; Walmsley, 2001). In this space, unlike in formal debates, we do not look for winners and losers; rather, it provides a medium for finding common ground, sometimes by addressing mistrust and misconceptions. While the network has indeed sought to make recommendations and decisions, dialogue provides the means to achieve consensus. Importantly, AfriNEAD is not responsible for doing research itself but rather for facilitating and coordinating an enabling environment for others to do research in relevant areas, helping to identify gaps and to fill them with useable ideas through dialogue and networking.

1.3.2 *Implement Research on Evidence-to-Action in Disability (READ) for Africa*

The AfriNEAD network intended to work with member countries to develop a methodology for profiling their own local situation regarding persons with disabilities, the services available to them, the research being conducted and areas needing investigation, and to identify facilitators and barriers for turning evidence into action. It is anticipated that countries will submit their 'state of our nation' analysis for publication in an e-book available on the AfriNEAD webpage www.sun.ac.za/webmail. This publication, entitled *Research on evidence-to-action in disability for Africa* (*READ for Africa*), will be an important advocacy document. The publication will act as a dissemination tool for the network's activities, will provide opportunities for researchers to contribute to a reputable forum of high status and will act as a mechanism to link with research support.

1.3.3 *Establish AfriNEAD Country Working Groups to Produce Best Evidence-to-Action Practice Guidelines*

AfriNEAD's aim was to establish interdisciplinary and multi-perspective 'working groups' tasked with identifying action pathways and producing best evidence-to-action practice guidelines which would be published on the AfriNEAD webpage. Work groups are essential platforms for dialogue and debates, thus engendering change processes with principles of participation, consensus building and joint decision-making within AfriNEAD. The approach allows 'cross-fertilisation' of ideas, reduced bias, increased risk taking, high commitment, improved communication and overall, we hope, achievement of better solutions. Each African country affiliated to AfriNEAD will develop roundtable discussion on disability research in their countries. This roundtable will constitute a similar structure as AfriNEAD constituting of a range of stakeholders as it is possible, including persons with disabilities, policymakers, practitioners and researchers and will use the UNCRPD to drive its research activities.

1.3.4 Host Triannual AfriNEAD Conferences

Another platform that was essential for the dissemination and utilization of research was the AfriNEAD conference, held at least once every three years. This three-day Africa-wide conference focuses on specified themes of interest to network members to assess progress on evidence-to-action and to consolidate and strengthen dialogue. The intention was to host the symposium on a rotation basis by member countries, with each event producing a collection of papers to be published as a special issue of a suitable international journal. The first special issue focusing on the 2007 AfriNEAD conference was published by the well-established international journal of *Disability and Rehabilitation.* A paper in the respected *Disability and Society* subsequently outlined the outcomes of the 2009 AfriNEAD Symposium (Mji et al., 2011). The *African Journal of Disability (AJOD)* is the second journal since the inauguration of AfriNEAD in 2007 to table a special issue focusing on the AfriNEAD Symposium. Indeed, the impetus for the AJOD comes from the enthusiasm generated by energetic researchers meeting through AfriNEAD.

1.3.5 Develop a Consortium Inclusive of Persons with Disabilities, Academic Researchers, Business, Government and Civil Society (DABGC)

There was a need to bridge the gap between all critical stakeholders of AfriNEAD. The desire for a mutual exchange of skills, knowledge and resources led to the development of a DABGC Consortium, linking disability, academia, business, government and civil society, proposed as a platform for engaging sectors of the consortium that have a direct impact on and association with the world of persons with disabilities. The proposed focus of the DABGC Consortium will be to address the gaps that exist between the stakeholders' worlds, especially those of business and people with disabilities—for instance by developing plans to facilitate the entry of qualified persons with disabilities into the workplace and supporting the vision and goals of AfriNEAD through use of combined resources. In the section below in Table 1.1 are organizations linked to the development of the DABGC:

Table 1.1 Organizations linked to the DABGC

South Africa	*Regional (In Africa but outside South Africa)*	*International*
Western Cape Network on Disabilities DeafNet—A network for knowledge and expertise of people in Africa of people with hearing loss and communication barriers. DPSA—Disabled People South Africa NID—National Institute for the Deaf DICAG—Disabled Children Action Group Cape Town Association for the Physically Disabled	SAFOD—Southern Africa Federation for the Disabled Secretariat of the African Decade for Persons with Disabilities (now African Disability Alliance) Kwame Nkrumah University of Science and Technology (KNUST) Centre for Social Studies, University of Malawi	SINTEF Norway Washington University Centre for Global Health, at Trinity College, Dublin, Ireland, Cheshire Homes and CBM and Enablement in the Netherlands KU Leuven University Belgium

AfriNEAD Business plan, 2021–2025

1.3.6 *Partnerships with Institutions of Higher Learning*

Through partnering with institutions of higher learning in Africa in creating Disability and Rehabilitation Programmes, AfriNEAD plays a supportive role in these programmes and fosters focus on development of disability research evidence and encourages translation of this evidence into policy and action for the realization of rights of persons with disabilities (Mji et al., 2011). For example, through AfriNEAD partnership with the DDRS, AfriNEAD assisted Kwame Nkrumah University of Science and Technology (KNUST) in Kumasi Ghana in establishing a postgraduate BSC programme in Disability and Rehabilitation Studies and a Masters in Disability Studies (Mji & Edusei, 2019). The two institutions have a memorandum of agreement stipulating that the DDRS will provide KNUST with ongoing support in strengthening the programmes (Mji & Edusei, 2019; AfriNEAD Business plan, 2021–2025).

1.4 AfriNEAD Governance

1.4.1 Organizational Structure

Initially the activities of AfriNEAD were governed by the Secretariat based at the DDRS and the Advisory Working Group. Later this structure was named the Governing Body with a Governing document that plays the role of a constitution (AfriNEAD Governance Document, 2022).

1.4.1.1 The Core/Advisory Working Group/Governing Body

An interim International Advisory Working Group was established in 2007 which gives strategic and practical advice on the projects and activities that AfriNEAD undertakes. As the network develops it was anticipated that each member country/region would be represented in the Advisory Working Group, which would be charged with approving the Annual Report of the network, approving budgetary management and control functions and generally steering the network to address such issues as research and policy priorities, emerging focus areas, and will pay urgent attention to the monitoring and evaluation of progress. A new group should be elected at each AfriNEAD conference (AfriNEAD Business Plan, 2019; Mji et al., 2009a).

1.4.1.2 Composition of the Advisory Working Group

Currently, the Advisory Working Group comprises of 25 members: 16 academics, seven representatives of DPOs, one disability activist and one from the business sector. The countries represented in the group are Botswana, Ghana, Norway, Malawi, United Kingdom, Ireland, Zambia and South Africa. The network is also making efforts in inviting more personnel from the business sector to be part of the Advisory Working Group (AfriNEAD Business Plan, 2019; Mji et al., 2009a). Since AfriNEAD was still supported by the Governing structure created in 2007, a new Governing structure consisting of three tier is being proposed as explained in Table 1.2:

Table 1.2 Proposed new Governing structure for AfriNEAD

The three tier of the new Governing structure for AfriNEAD
A. 1st Tier of Governing structure of AfriNEAD: Management structure of AfriNEAD: These were the people that assisted: • with the presentation of 2023, 7th AfriNEAD conference • and will support AfriNEAD secretariat at the Division of Disability and Rehabilitation studies **B. 2nd Tier of Governing structure of AfriNEAD: Disability Research Country Working Groups (DRCWGs):** • These are the disability research working groups based in countries affiliated to AfriNEAD • They join the AfriNEAD management meetings to learn more about the functioning of AfriNEAD **C. The 3rd Tier of AfriNEAD:** • Are retired governing members of AfriNEAD and will sit in the Governing Structure of AfriNEAD for advisory purposes • They will join the AfriNEAD meetings twice a year. (AfriNEAD Governance document, 2022)

1.5 Challenges Remaining

1.5.1 Financial Constraints

AfriNEAD has been sustained mainly by funds raised towards running conferences which have not been enough to expand the activities of the network. There is a general lack of funds to cater for the day-to-day running costs of the AfriNEAD Secretariat and to expand human resources. The lack of human resources posed limits to what the network could achieve in the past sixteen years, especially in the planning and organization of conferences and supporting Disability Country Working Groups (DRCWGs).

1.5.2 Location

The location of the AfriNEAD Secretariat at the DDRS at Stellenbosch University is questioned by some persons with disabilities who feel that it implies a pure academic agenda and hence it should be dissociated from the university premises. This is something that the Secretariat and the Advisory Group have continuously reflected upon and concluded that the location is suitable given the agenda of AfriNEAD and the role that the

DDRS and Stellenbosch University, Stellenbosch, South Africa, play in the sustenance of AfriNEAD.

1.5.3 *Relationships*

Initially, AfriNEAD was challenged with the need to bridge the gap between researchers who were viewed as 'experts' and persons with disabilities who were viewed as outsiders. Ongoing dialogue amongst the different stakeholders has had a far-reaching impact in bridging this gap, although efforts to build relationships of mutual trust remain an ongoing process.

1.5.4 *Disability Research Country Working Groups*

Establishment of operational Disability Research Country Working Groups (DRCWGs) is still work in progress that requires a more focused and robust approach and workforce to steer it. There is a need for continuous support from the scientific committee through maintaining contact with the DRCWGs, monitoring their progress and offering guidance where necessary. A more detailed account of DRCWGs is presented in Chapter 7.

1.5.5 *Keeping Research Focused*

AfriNEAD is working towards keeping research agenda streamlined and focused to have an impact on policy and practice at a given time. For example, the target for 2021–2225 was to focus on assistive technology and its central role in emancipation of persons with disabilities in concord with the global WHO GATE Project. Assistive technology is a basic need for most persons with disabilities to be able to participate in all facets of society. Hence, AfriNEAD, as a custodian of disability research and partnerships on the African continent, decided to facilitate research around assistive technology which will provide evidence and guidelines for African States in ensuring that basic assistive devices are available and affordable for persons with disabilities in their countries. AfriNEAD will seek the support and collaboration of the African Union (AU) so that the research agenda may be prioritized on the African development/transformative agenda (AfriNEAD Business Plan, 2019; Mji et al., 2011).

1.6 Monitoring and Evaluation

Since its inception, AfriNEAD has used a reflective way of monitoring and evaluating its activities. The Governing Body meets twice per year to discuss and reflect on pertinent issues and at every AfriNEAD Conference there is a special meeting of the Governing Body that reflects on what worked well and what did not as well as how things can be improved in the future. The members are also kept informed of the activities of the network through a quarterly newspaper which is emailed to all of them.

Going into the future, AfriNEAD will identify and establish performance indicators for its planned outcomes and outputs. As activities become more formalized, a performance management plan will be put in place and updated as needed. All AfriNEAD projects and activities will be evaluated at biannual general meetings when the plan is established (AfriNEAD Business Plan, 2019).

1.7 Overview of Chapters

The intention of this book is to present a tapestry of AfriNEAD as it attempts to fulfil its quest of being a disability research network in the African region. The book covers ten chapters that are interrelated. In trying to develop links between chapters, there is some repetition on information already presented in previous chapters. Below is the overview of chapters that are covered by the book:

Chapter 1: The Quest to Develop an African Disability Research Network: in this first chapter the rationale and aims and objectives for developing AfriNEAD is outlined.

Chapter 2: "Nothing about us without us": Persons with disabilities' active participation in the development of AfriNEAD: the second chapter presents the contribution made by persons with disabilities in the development of AfriNEAD.

Chapter 3: The African Network for Evidence-to-Action in Disability: A role player in the realization of the UNCRPD in Africa: this chapter outlines how AfriNEAD used the UNCRPD as a prong to drive its disability research agenda.

Chapter 4: AfriNEAD considerations and response in conducting ethical driven disability research: this chapter presents some considerations given by AfriNEAD researchers and practitioners in addressing some of the ethical dilemmas in disability research.

Chapter 5: AfriNEAD conferences: AfriNEAD conferences have been one of the important networking platforms since AfriNEAD inauguration in 2007, this chapter outlines the process and outcome of presenting AfriNEAD conferences.

Chapter 6: The contribution of AfriNEAD to Disability Research in Africa: this chapter outlines how AfriNEAD has started to contribute to disability research in Africa.

Chapter 7: The Development of Disability Research Country Working Groups: this chapter presents an AfriNEAD strategy on how to link with countries associated with AfriNEAD to ensure that AfriNEAD approaches and concepts are implemented in these countries.

Chapter 8: African perspective on disability: this chapter presents how disability debates and scholarship is mainly influenced by thinking from the Global North and the need to decolonize disability debates in Africa.

Chapter 9: The guidance of African thinking to assist AfriNEAD achieve sustainability: this chapter presents how AfriNEAD has achieved sustainability by using African thinking.

Chapter 10: The Future of Disability Research in Africa: This final chapter draws research outcomes from previous conferences to suggest and map out a path for disability research in the region.

1.8 Chapter Conclusion

Given the history of exclusion and oppression of persons with disabilities in the region, many disability activists are suspicious of and hostile towards the entire research enterprise. The struggle of persons with disabilities in Africa is complicated by an absence of African understanding of disability (Mji et al., 2011). There is a general concern that Western theories with definitions rooted in the medical model of disability are generally promoted internationally in regions such as Africa (Bezzina, 2018; Mji, 2012). The quest for AfriNEAD to be a sustainable Network is not easy (Mji et al., 2009a). AfriNEAD has achieved its resilience by drawing from the collective conscious of Ubuntu and other African concepts and principles such as "uhambo Aluqgitwa ngemini enye—a journey is not finished in one day", "Ubude Abuphangwa—You cannot hurry to be tall" (Bergh, 2017; Boon, 1996; Chikane, 2012). These African concepts will be discussed in detail in subsequent chapters. The next chapter presents the contribution made by persons with disabilities in the development of AfriNEAD.

References

AfriNEAD conferences reports. (2007, 2009, 20211, 2014, 2017, 2020 & 2023). www.sun.ac.za/AfriNEAD

AfriNEAD Governance Document. (2022). www.sun.ac.za/AfriNEAD

AfriNEAD Business plan. (2019). *2021–2025 AfriNEAD Secretariat*. Stellenbosch University, Stellenbosch.

Balton, S., Arvidsson, P., Granlund, M., Huus, K., & Dada, S. (2021). Test-retest reliability of Picture My participation in children with intellectual disability in South Africa. *Scandinavian Journal of occupational Therapy, 29*(4), 315–324. https://doi.org/10. 1080/11038128.2020.1856922

Barnes, C., & Mercer, G. (Eds.). (1997). *Doing disability research*. University of Leeds, Disability Press.

Bergh, M. (2017). Practices and discourses of Ubuntu: Implications for an African model of disability. *African Journal of Disability, 6*, 292.

Bezzina, L. (2018). The role of indigenous and external knowledge in development interventions with disabled people in Burkina Faso: The implications of engaging with lived experiences. *Disability and the Global South, 5*(2), 1488–1507.

Boon, M. (1996). *The African way. The power of interactive leadership*. Struik Publishers.

Charlton, J. I. (1998). Nothing about us without us. University of California Press–Social Sciences.

Chikane, F. (2012). Eight days in September: The removal of Thabo Mbeki. Johannesburg, South Africa: Picador Africa.

Dragon, S. S., Mobus, N., Beck, S., Stang, E. M., Mobhlenkamp, S., Joeckel, K. H., Erbe, l. R., & Siegrist, J. (2008, May). Low socio-economic positions are associated with poor social networks and social support: Results from the Heinz Nixdorf Recall Study. *International Journal for Equity in Health, 5,* 7:13.

Friedman, S. R., Mateu-Gelabert, P., Curtis, R., Maslow, C., Bolyard, M., Sandoval, M., & Flom, P. L. (2007, June). Social capital or networks, negotiations, and norms? Neighbourhood case study. *Am J Prev. Med., 32* (6 Supplement),: S160–70.

Howell, C., Chalklen, S., & Alberts, T. (2006). A history of disability rights in South Africa. In B. Watermeyer, L. Swartz, T. Lorenzo, & M. Priestley (Eds.), *Disability and Social Change South African Agenda*. HSRC.

Ingstad, B., & Whyte, S. R. (2007). Disability connections. In B. Ingstad & S. R. Whyte (Eds.), *Disability in Local and Global Worlds*. University of California Press.

Kachaje, R., Dube, K., MacLachlan, M., & Mji, G. (2014). The African network for evidence-to-action on disability: A role player in the realisation of the UNCRPD in Africa. *AJOD, 3* (2).

MacLachlan, M., Mji, G., Chataika, T., Wazakili, M., Dube, A. K., Mulumba, M., Massah, B., Wakene, D., Kallon, F., & Maughan, M. (2014). Facilitating disability inclusion in poverty reduction processes: Group consensus perspectives from disability stakeholders in Uganda, Malawi, Ethiopia, and Sierra Leone *Disability and the Global South, OPEN ACCESS,* Vol. 1, No. 1, 107–127 ISSN 2050–7364 www.dgsjournal.org

Mji, G. (2012). *The health knowledge utilised by rural older Xhosa women in the management of health problems in their home situation, with a special focus on indigenous knowledge [Doctoral Thesis]*. University of Stellenbosch.

Mji, G., MacLachlan, M., Melling-Williams, N., & Gcaza, S. (2009a). Realising the Rights of disabled people in Africa: An introduction to the special issue. *Disability and Rehabilitation, 31*(1), 1–6.

Mji, G., Gcaza, S., Melling–Williams, N., MacLachlan, M. (2009b). Networking in disability for development: Introducing the African network for evidence-to- action on disability. In M. MacLachlan & L. Swartz (Eds.), Disability, and international development towards inclusive global health. Springer, pp. 69–89.

Mji, G., Gcaza, S., Swartz, L., MacLachlan, M., Hutton, B. (2011). An African way of networking around disability. *Disability and Society; 26*(3).

Mji, G., & Edusei, A. (2019). 'An introduction to a special issue on the role of assistive technology in social inclusion of persons with disabilities in Africa: Outcome of the fifth African network for evidence-to-action in disability conference. *African Journal of Disability, 8*(0), a681. https://doi. org/ https://doi.org/10.4102/AJOD. v8i0.681

Panda, S. (2024). *Leaving No One behind: Achieving the Sustainable Development Goals through Accessibility for People with Disabilities International Journal of Educational Communications and Technology (IJECT), 4*(1), 16–26.

South African Integrated National Disability Strategy White Paper. (1997). Retrieved 7 August, 2023, from http://www.info.gov.za/whitepapers/1997/ disability.htm

South African Employment Equity Act. (1998). Retrieved 7 August, 2023, from http://www.labourguide.co.za/EE.pdf

Swartz, L. (2014). Five challenges for disability-related research in sub-Saharan Africa. *African Journal of Disability, 3*(2), 149.

Strnadová, I., Dowse, L., & Garcia-Lee, B. (2022). *Doing research inclusively: Co-production inaction*, Disability Innovation Institute, UNSW, Sydney.

Tilley, E., Strnadová, I., Ledger, S., Walmsley, J., Loblinzk, J., Christian, P. A., et al. (2021). "Working together is like a partnership of entangled knowledge": Exploring the sensitivities of doing participatory data analysis with people with learning disabilities. *International Journal of Social Research Methodology, 24*(5), 567–579. https://doi.org/10.1080/13645579.2020.1857970

United Nations. (2006). *Convention on the rights of persons with disabilities.* Retrieved 7 August, 2023, from https://www.ohchr.org/en/instruments-mechanisms/instruments/convention-rights-persons-disabilities

Walmsley, J. (2001). *Normalisation, Emancipatory Research and Inclusive Research in Learning Disability, Disability & Society, 16*(2), 187–205. 10.101080/09687590120035807

CHAPTER 2

"Nothing About Us Without Us": Persons with Disabilities' Active Participation in the Development of AfriNEAD

Gubela Mji and Washiela Sait

2.1 Introduction

This chapter presents the active participation of persons with disabilities in the development of AfriNEAD and the lessons learnt by AfriNEAD from the existing networks of persons with disabilities. From its inception in 2007, AfriNEAD had an ambitious agenda of being an inclusive network drawing on the best skills, expertise and goodwill of researchers and disability activists. One of the key stakeholders that AfriNEAD intended to include as key drivers of the network was persons with disabilities. Individuals with disabilities have demonstrated significant resilience and networking abilities, leading to notable advancements in disability-related issues. Among their accomplishments is the publication of foundational

G. Mji (✉) · W. Sait
Cape Town, South Africa
e-mail: gumji@sun.ac.za

W. Sait
e-mail: banienw@gmail.com

G. Mji (ed.), *Doing Disability Research in Africa*,
https://doi.org/10.1007/978-3-031-98549-2_2

works on disability, which have contributed to shaping the discourse and understanding of disability studies (Howell et al., 2006).

A pivotal moment in disability advocacy was the walkout by persons with disabilities from the Rehabilitation International (RI) conference in Winnipeg, Canada, in 1980, which led to the establishment of Disability International (DI) (Howell et al., 2006). This action marked a significant challenge to the prevailing dominance of health professionals in shaping the disability agenda (Howell et al., 2006). More recently, individuals with disabilities played a critical role in the development of the United Nations Convention on the Rights of Persons with Disabilities (UNCRPD), which, since its adoption in 2008, has been integrated into international law. Their contributions have had profound implications both morally and practically, outlining essential steps for realizing the rights of persons with disabilities (Kachaje et al., 2014; Phiri, 2014).

The slogan 'Nothing About Us Without Us' encapsulates the core philosophy and historical trajectory of the Disability Rights Movement (DRM). This movement has pursued a mission that parallels the broader liberation struggles against oppression, with a particular emphasis on autonomy and self-determination. At the heart of the DRM's advocacy is a relentless demand for control over the policies and decisions that affect the lives of persons with disabilities. This theme of control is not merely a rhetorical device but a critical response to the systemic conditions that have historically rendered individuals with disabilities powerless. These conditions—characterized by enforced dependency, pervasive poverty, societal degradation and institutionalization—have long dictated the lived experiences of persons with disabilities (Charlton, 1998).

This entrenched dependency, often reinforced by paternalistic attitudes, begins typically at the onset of disability and persists throughout the individual's life, culminating only in death. Such a condition is not an isolated phenomenon but is, in fact, a reality for hundreds of millions of people across the globe. It is only within the last twenty-five years that we have witnessed a significant shift in this narrative, driven primarily by the efforts of persons with disabilities themselves. Although this transformation has occurred on a relatively small scale and has impacted only a fraction of the global disabled population, its implications are profound. This emerging change challenges long-standing paradigms of disability and dependency, signalling a gradual but pivotal reconfiguration of the social and political landscape for individuals with disabilities (Ned et al., 2022).

In the early stages of disability research within academia, the focus on adult disability largely excluded considerations of children with disabilities and the broader impact of disability on families. At that time, research on childhood disability was predominantly clinical, emphasizing impairment rather than the lived experiences of children and their families (Philpott & Sait, 2009). However, the emergence of a parent-led movement Disabled Children Action Group (DiCaG) advocating for the human rights and equality of children with disabilities and drawing inspiration from the adult disability rights movement has played a significant role in shifting academic attention towards childhood disability. This movement catalysed a more holistic approach to research, incorporating the perspectives of children with disabilities and their families into the academic discourse (Philpott & Sait, 2009).

The engagement of adults with disabilities and parents of children with disabilities has facilitated the development of robust research networks that prioritize disability and human rights, ensuring that academic discourses are grounded in real-world experiences and challenges. Through activism and sustained advocacy, persons with disabilities have challenged traditional power dynamics within academia, advocating for methodologies that respect and amplify their voices. This has led to more equitable and participatory research practices, which in turn have influenced policy and practice on a national scale (Botha & Ohajunwa, 2024).

These gains achieved by persons with disabilities in highlighting the plight of persons with disabilities as a human right and a development issue, illustrated during the early days of development of AfriNEAD the sophisticated networking skills of persons with disabilities. In this chapter we will present how AfriNEAD learnt from the experience of disability networks and persons with disabilities in the quest to be a regional research network for evidence to action in disability. The next section presents on how AfriNEAD drew experiences in networking from the disability rights movement.

2.2 Drawing Experiences in Networking from the Disability Rights Movement (DRM)

Individuals with disabilities have demonstrated remarkable resilience and strategic networking, leading to significant achievements within the disability rights movement. A pivotal accomplishment was the formation of the Union of the Physically Impaired Against Segregation (UPIAS) in 1976, a landmark organization that profoundly influenced the discourse on disability. The UPIAS's publication of the "Fundamental Principles of Disability" played a critical role in shaping the theoretical foundation of disability studies, shifting the focus from a medicalized view of disability to one that recognizes the social and structural barriers faced by people with disabilities (Howell et al., 2006).

One of their core statements was related to the acknowledgement of the role that society plays in further disabling persons with disabilities, when they stated that:

> In our view it is society which disables physically impaired people. Disability is something imposed on top of our impairments by the way we are unnecessarily isolated and excluded from full participation in society (Howell et al., 2006: 49).

During that time, persons with disabilities began challenging the dominance of health professionals in shaping the disability agenda. The establishment of Disabled Peoples' International (DPI) spurred significant global initiatives that opposed the marginalization and oppression of persons with disabilities. One such initiative was the United Nations' declaration of 1981 as the International Year of Disabled Persons (IYPD). This was followed by the World Programme of Action Concerning Disabled Persons, which provided a universal framework for addressing discrimination and promoting equal opportunities worldwide. Subsequently, the Decade of Disabled Persons (1982–1992) led to the formulation of the Standard Rules on the Equalization of Opportunities for People with Disabilities and contributed to the growth of Disabled Persons' Organizations (DPOs) (Howell et al., 2006: 49).

The UN Convention on the Rights of Persons with Disabilities (United Nations, 2006), which entered international law in 2008, represents one of the most significant steps—both morally and practically—towards realizing the rights of persons with disabilities. The Convention aims to address discrimination, change perceptions and combat stereotypes and prejudices towards persons with disabilities. Article 32 of the Convention emphasizes that countries must provide development assistance to support developing nations in implementing the Convention (United Nations, 2006). This article places a dual responsibility on high-income countries: they must not only implement the Convention domestically but also ensure that their efforts help to put it into action in low-income countries, thereby ensuring that no one is left behind (Panda, 2024).

These achievements by persons with disabilities, which highlight their struggles with both human rights and development issues, underscore the sophisticated networking skills they have employed to confront and overcome years of discrimination and oppression (Mji et al., 2009a, b).

The formation of the African Disability Forum (ADF) conceived during a Consultative Meeting on November 28–29, 2012, at the UN Conference Centre in Addis Ababa, Ethiopia, brought attention to African lived realities and experiences of disability. Organized by the UN Special Rapporteur on Disability, with support from the UN Department of Economic and Social Affairs (DESA) and the UN Economic Commission for Africa (UNECA), the meeting brought together African disability organizations, academic institutions and development partners. Participants endorsed the initiative to establish ADF as a DPO-led organization dedicated to advancing the rights and inclusion of persons with disabilities across Africa. This initiative gained urgency following the adoption of the African Union's "Disability Architecture" (AUDA) by the AU Conference of Ministers of Social Development in November 2012. Supported by a grant from the Abilis Foundation, a planning meeting in December 2013 solidified the ADF's organizational structure and priorities. The ADF was formally launched on November 17–19, 2014, in Addis Ababa, with regional and national DPO leaders in attendance. The first ADF General Assembly, held on October 31-November 1, 2015, at the Desmond Tutu Conference Centre in Nairobi, Kenya, marked a historic moment as Africa established its first democratic, representative regional disability forum, culminating in the adoption of the ADF Constitution and Bylaws and the election of the inaugural Executive Council.

Table 2.1 presents some examples of international and national disability networks. These networks have been built up over many decades and are to be found in Africa at national, regional and global levels.

Table 2.1 shows how persons with disabilities have united as a collective to fight the discrimination that they have experienced and to regain their rights and human dignity.

Table 2.1 Examples of disability networks

Organization	*Membership*	*Goals*
Disabled Peoples International (DPI)	National organizations or assemblies of disabled people. A majority of the members as well as the Governing Body are persons with disabilities. Representatives to include all races, sex, religion, language, geography, etc.	To promote the human rights of disabled people through full participation, equalization of opportunity and development To promote the economic and social integration of disabled persons To develop and support organizations of disabled persons
Christian Blind Mission (CBM)	International, 700 partner organizations in developing countries throughout the world	To improve the quality of life of the world's poorest persons with disabilities and those at risk of disability in the most disadvantaged societies To support and develop local partner organizations, rather than implement projects To transfer knowledge and skills, both professional and managerial to development of these partners
Handicap International CAHD rebranded as Humanity & Inclusion as of 2018—Community Approaches to Handicap in Development	International, 55 countries worldwide	Focus on the causes of impairment, disability and handicap and the link to able-bodied people To create social change and inclusion as citizens with equal opportunities and full access to participation

(continued)

Table 2.1 (continued)

Organization	*Membership*	*Goals*
African Community-based Rehabilitation Network (CAN)	Based in Uganda Disabled persons in Africa and their families	To benchmark best practices and research about disability To make information about disability issues accessible worldwide through conferences, writer's workshops, the formation of CBR national organizations, maintaining a website and publishing To promote the equalization of opportunities, social integration and rehabilitation of persons with disabilities in Africa

(continued)

Table 2.1 (continued)

Organization	*Membership*	*Goals*
Southern Africa Federation for the Disabled (SAFOD)	16 countries within the Southern African Development Corporation (SADAC) region are affiliated to SAFOD	(i) Encouragement of the formation of organizations of disabled people in Southern Africa (ii) Provision of support and strengthening of existing affiliates (iii) Training of personnel and leaders of organizations of disabled people (iv) Promotion, support and complementing of government policies and programmes in favour of disabled people in the SADC region (v) Facilitation of information exchange as well as affiliation and cooperation with other regional, continental and international organizations

(continued)

Table 2.1 (continued)

Organization	*Membership*	*Goals*
Global Partnership for Disability and Development (GPDD)	International, persons with disabilities and their families, including those born with disabilities and those disabled through wars, violence, traffic or work injuries, disease, disasters and other causes	To accelerate the inclusion of persons with disabilities and their families into development policies and practices To increase collaboration among development agencies and organizations to reduce the extreme poverty and exclusion of a substantial number of children, women and men with disabilities who are living in poor countries
The Secretariat of the African Decade of Persons with Disabilities (SADPD)	Africa, governments, Decade Steering Committees (DSCs), Disabled Persons' Organisations (DPOs), development organizations	To empower African organizations to work in partnership to include disability issues and persons with disabilities in policies and programmes in all sectors of society in Africa To strengthen DSCs in at least 20 African countries by 2009 To assist the most vulnerable disability groups, e.g. persons with mental disabilities, deaf, or blind persons, persons with albinism to build strong African DPOs

Mji et al. (2009a, b)

2.3 Challenges Still Facing Disability Networking and Disability Rights Movement

Despite numerous progressive statements and initiatives in recent years, meaningful improvements in the quality of life for persons with disabilities in Africa remain limited (Mji, 2009a). The historical exclusion of persons with disabilities from full participation in society persists, highlighting the need for more substantial change and social development to achieve a truly inclusive society (Mji, 2009a). As shown in Table 2.1 there are many networks that have been developed by persons with disabilities to fight for their human rights and dignity. The challenge with these networks is sustainability. Availability of continuous funding remains a problem that undermines the development and completion of ideas as most funding comes from international bodies that have a funding tenure. This results in lack of build-up and development of ideas that could be turned into action for the realization of rights for persons with disabilities within the African region. It is in this regard that AfriNEAD advocated for an inclusive network that includes, persons with disabilities, academics, business, government and civil society formations. It is envisaged that challenges facing networking for the rights of persons with disabilities including how to fund disability networks could be discussed as a collective with the hope of creating sustainable solutions.

2.4 Persons with Disabilities and Their Standpoint on Matters That Are About Them

The World report on disability (WHO, 2011) outlines the development of a social model of disability, largely through the efforts of persons with disabilities in reaction to the medicalization of disability by health professionals. Different 'models' of disability have been positioned as being dichotomous, thereby stifling dialogue about the relative impact of impairment and environment (Grue, 2011). The International Classification of Functioning, Disability and Health (ICF) is presented in the World report on disability as a framework that can begin to bridge this gap, recognizing both the nature of impairment and the importance of environmental factors. The environmental factors within the life-situation of a person with an impairment may either pose barriers or be a facilitator to participation (WHO, 2002). Within the UNCRPD, such barriers are seen as a form of social injustice that states have an obligation to address (UN, 2006). For Barnes (2008), an emancipatory research approach must at least include a focus on environmental barriers and must prioritize the knowledge and experience of persons with disabilities.

The involvement of persons with disabilities in disability research can be seen as existing along a continuum, ranging from weak to strong engagement. At the weak end of the scale, involvement would be in the form of researchers engaging with persons with disabilities merely as subjects of research or perhaps for consultation at an advanced stage of research. At the strong end of the scale, disabled people's organisations (DPOs) would be involved in setting the research agenda as well as in conducting, commissioning and disseminating the research. This was found to be true in a specific European context; among persons with disabilities there was 'in particular, a desire to be involved in shaping research agendas and defining research questions whilst valuing the methodological expertise and credibility of academic researchers' (Priestley et al., 2010: 741).

Research ownership is a highly contested issue, with Disabled Persons' Organizations (DPOs) frequently criticizing academic researchers for using their work primarily for career advancement rather than for the genuine empowerment of persons with disabilities (Garbutt & Seymour, 1998). Carmichael (2004) emphasizes that research should be a means to an end, driving action rather than merely serving as an academic exercise. To be truly effective, research must be communicated in ways that translate into tangible outcomes, rather than gathering dust on a shelf. In the southern African context, Chalklen, Seutloadi, and Sadek (2009) found that disability research often lacks a solution-oriented focus and fails to provide actionable material for advocacy, as it is frequently too generic. Moreover, the lack of disaggregated statistics renders the data less useful for disability activists. Addressing these criticisms is crucial if researchers are to contribute meaningfully to the empowerment of persons with disabilities, as envisioned in Article 31 of the UNCRPD (McKenzie et al., 2014).

2.5 The Role of Persons with Disabilities in Building Communities of Trust in AfriNEAD

In 2011, AfriNEAD held its third conference in Victoria Falls, Zimbabwe, under the theme 'Building Communities of Trust in Disability Research '. This theme arose from the recognition that, despite extensive discussions during the previous two AfriNEAD conferences about the importance of collaboration between persons with disabilities and disability researchers, a significant level of mistrust persisted between these groups. In this section, we honour the contributions of two remarkable disability activists, Dr Rachel Kachaje and Mr Alexander Mwanza Phiri, both of whom are no longer with us. Their voices were instrumental in advancing the dialogue on the inclusion of persons with disabilities in disability research. Notably, Mr Phiri's paper, prepared for this conference, was presented posthumously (Phiri, 2014). We acknowledge their enduring legacy and the vital role they played in bridging the gap between researchers and the disability community. Below under 2.5.1 is the keynote address presented by Dr Rachel Kachaje in the 2011 AfriNEAD conference.

2.5.1 Partnership in Disability Research—A Vehicle for Achieving Equality for Persons with Disabilities

"I have been involved with Southern Africa Federation of the Disabled (SAFOD) for many years. Before that, I used to attend different workshops as an ordinary delegate from my country until in 2002 when I changed the course of history to become the first woman to successfully head the organisation. The secret to that success was that, when I was elected as chairperson, I immediately realized that I had shouldered a heavy responsibility which I did not have the capacity to manage alone. So, what I did was to look around me and identified the gaps that I have in my knowledge and looked where I could get the expertise to fill up those gaps.

When I identified the expertise and talent to fill up the gaps for the area of my responsibility, I felt very comfortable knowing that I had some partnerships to help me achieve my objective of taking SAFOD to another higher level. So, if there are any success stories about SAFOD during my tenure of office, this was the secret, I was tapping on the talent, knowledge, skills and expertise from different partners that I had identified. I am also reminded of the process on producing the UNCRPD. There were many players and voices that were united as if there was one voice. We had one aim, purpose and one objective. Through this process, the International Disability Caucus (IDC) was formed.

Disability rights activists from across the world, have followed closely on the development of this landmark treaty, and waited with abated breath as the Convention proceeded through the different processes and stages in the UN system—from the negotiations to the adoption and opening for signature on the 30th of March 2007, and finally, its entry into force on the 3rd of May.

Rights based approaches required the full participation of all relevant stakeholders; in this case the CRPD required that governments consult with persons with disabilities and their representative organisations in issues that affected their lives. You know the slogan "Nothing about us, without us" in other words nothing about disabled without the disabled. If you have heard about the "them and us" or "theirs and ours" scenarios, they arise out of lack of partnerships or lack of participation.

So, what would society miss out on if they do not include persons with disabilities? They will miss out on a large pool of talent. Few people realize that 'Disability is not inability'. Many people, including some doctors, don't know that to have a "twisted body does not mean to have a twisted brain'. Persons with disabilities can contribute significantly to a wide array of expertise, skills and talents in many development agendas. Responding to the voices of persons with disabilities when we develop the partnerships which are geared towards developing an equitable world" (Kachaje in the 2011, AfriNEAD conference).

2.5.2 *Persons with Disabilities Have Got to Lead the Experience of Being Disabled*

Mr Alexander Mwanza Phiri prepared a keynote address for the 2011 AfriNEAD conference and he died before presenting this paper. The paper was converted into a publication and below is a piece extracted from that paper:

"I can go on and on asking questions, which is, in fact, what most researchers spend their time doing, often writing volumes of text in the process but finding very few, and sometimes no useful, answers to their questions. I am not saying that people, or researchers for that matter, should not ask questions and try to find answers to these questions. Researchers need to set questions and indeed work on the solutions; but as they do so, I believe they need to reach out and work together. We need to respect one another's environment; we need to respect each other's situation and position. There may be distinctions in terms of who we are, where we live or where we come from; what position we hold in society; whether we are in or outside government; whether we are black or white; have a disability or not—we need to find a way of working together because the essence of life is that every human being is important. Each institution is important in its own way; hence the need for all of us to work together in our pursuit of the research agenda. We need to support one another.

Recognizing the important role of researchers, it is now the time to develop the capacity of researchers with disabilities. This is, in fact, what we are aiming to achieve through a new initiative that we have started with the support of the United Kingdom's Department for International Development (DFID). The SAFOD Research Programme (SRP) is teaching us that people with disabilities are the best to tell their own story and to drive their own research agenda.

Through the SRP we have also learnt that collaboration in the research process is important not only for capacity building but also for effective engagement with academia and mainstream researchers. The idea is to not let persons with disabilities continue as passengers on the research train; they must be in the engine room and steer that train.

Regarding the SRP, the criterion set by the Technical Advisory Board (TAB) that each bidder should have a person with disability as part of the research team is not merely to say people with disability should be used as window dressing. Instead, we want them to participate fully because they will soon be driving this process. To achieve this, however, we need to ensure that collaborative efforts between organizations in developed and developing countries yield mutual benefits. This must be achieved through genuinely equal (but not necessarily equivalent) partnerships; even though much of Africa does not have financial, technical and material resources, Africa does have a wealth of talented people, and this resource does and should include persons with disabilities. Much more research on disability issues is needed for positive and effective policy development in Africa. (Phiri, 2014)".

2.5.3 *Key Points Emerging from the Presentations of Dr Kachaje and the Paper of Mr Phiri*

The voices of Dr Kachaje and Mr Phiri underscore the critical importance of partnership in disability research, viewing it as an interdependent endeavour. They emphasize that collaboration not only enhances the quality of research but also accelerates its completion. Both advocates strongly for the development of partnerships in disability research, a perspective that has been integral to the establishment of the African Network for Evidence to Action in Disability (AfriNEAD). This network aims to bridge gaps across various issues relevant to realizing the rights of people with disabilities (Mji et al., 2009a, b). A key motivation for AfriNEAD's creation was to assess the quality and relevance of existing disability research. The network highlights a clear challenge: it is not merely the quantity of research that needs to be increased, but its quality, and more importantly, its ability to be translated into effective policy and practice. Translating research into evidence-based advocacy, policy, practice and products—especially within the pan-African context—requires systematic coordination that is coherent, consistent and collaborative. Only through such an approach can research evidence serve as a catalyst for advancing human rights instruments like the UNCRPD (Mji et al., 2009a, b). Central to this coordinated effort are the lived experiences of persons with disabilities and their families who must take the lead in sharing their stories and shaping the research agenda. The following section will explore the contributions of disability organizations to the development of AfriNEAD.

2.6 The Contribution of Disability Organizations to the Development of AfriNEAD

2.6.1 Summary of the Development and Intention of AfriNEAD

African Network for Evidence-to-Action in Disability (AfriNEAD) is a pan-African network founded by the Division of Disability and Rehabilitation Studies at Stellenbosch University in 2007. The network promotes, facilitates and coordinates implementation of disability research evidence into policy and practice through engaging persons with disabilities; researching with them, not only about them; and, where possible, making them, the lead researchers. This is achieved through: collaborative research projects involving persons with disabilities, academic researchers, government officials, business and civil society. Research evidence is disseminated using conferences, seminars, policy briefs, reports, publications and special issues in academic journals (Mji et al., 2009a, b; Phiri, 2014; Kachaje, 2014).

Numerous networks exist, each performing distinct functions. For a network to be truly beneficial to its members, it is crucial that these members are not only aware of the network's objectives but also understand that it operates with a specific approach tailored to a defined purpose. The proposed network aimed to include representatives from as many African countries as possible, and within each country, to encompass a diverse range of stakeholders. A key element of this inclusivity was the central involvement of persons with disabilities. AfriNEAD benefited from the fact that during the conception of an inclusive regional disability research network, several significant developments, linked to the progress made by persons with disabilities and the broader Disability Movement, were simultaneously unfolding and maturing. These developments and their contributions to the evolution of AfriNEAD are outlined below.

2.6.2 *The Contribution of the Southern Africa Federation for the Disabled (SAFOD) in the Development of AfriNEAD*

During the consolidation of the regional disability research network, we were fortunate to have the support of the Disabled People South Africa (DPSA) office in Cape Town, which connected us to its regional counterpart, the Southern Africa Federation for the Disabled (SAFOD). At that time, SAFOD was implementing the "SAFOD Research Programme (SRP)", a significant initiative aimed at gathering, compiling and disseminating information on the status of disability within the SADC region. The SRP, initially planned as a five-year program from 2007 to 2012, was funded by the Department for International Development (DfID). It encompassed a series of studies titled "Living Conditions of Persons with Disabilities in Southern Africa", along with the Disability Policy Audit and the DPO Needs Assessment.

Tragically, the lead of this program and SAFOD Chairperson, Mr Alexandria Mwanza Phiri, passed away in May 2011. Mr Phiri, who also served on the AfriNEAD Governing Body and attended its conferences in 2007 and 2009, was a strong advocate for the development of AfriNEAD and the African Journal of Disability (AJOD). He recommended Prof. Leslie Swartz as its Editor in Chief at the 2009 AfriNEAD Annual General Meeting (AGM). Under Mr Phiri's leadership, numerous research projects were funded by SAFOD and conducted by AfriNEAD researchers. During a Department for International Development (DfID) evaluation of the SRP who were the funders of the SRP, evaluators noted the overlap between AfriNEAD's work and that of the SRP. This alignment was no coincidence; both initiatives shared a common goal: the realization of the rights of persons with disabilities in Africa. Consequently, the efforts of these two research entities naturally converged.

2.6.3 *African Decade for Persons with Disabilities*

The African Decade of Persons with Disabilities (ADPD) was launched in 1999. This was an African-Union-declared effort to raise awareness about disability issues in the region and to identify solutions tailored to the African experience that enhanced full participation, equality and empowerment of Africans with disability. It was an initiative of the non-governmental community of Africa, in cooperation with member states and governments of the African Union (*formerly called the Organization of African Unity*), that is designed to increase inclusion of disabled Africans in poverty reduction programmes, increase the number of disabled children and youth in African schools and educational programmes and increase the numbers of disabled Africans receiving adequate health services. While originally expected to last until 2009, ADDP was extended for another 10 years (2010–2019) at a meeting held in Windhoek, Namibia, in October 2008 by African Union (AU) ministers in charge of social development.

The work that was conducted by the African Decade is now done by the African Disability Alliance under the leadership of Mr AK Dube. Mr Dube was Central to the Development of AfriNEAD. He sits within the Governing structure of AfriNEAD. When the SRP program was implemented by SAFOD, the African Decade became central to the implementation of the SRP programs and the development of AfriNEAD. Two projects come to mind when thinking of the relationship between AfriNEAD and the Decade and these are: the writing of the research manual for persons with disabilities—this research manual for persons with disabilities was commissioned by the Decade for AfriNEAD to develop. Other AfriNEAD related projects were the African Policy on Disability and development whereby the Decade in partnership with AfriNEAD and Trinity College explored the inclusion of persons with disabilities in poverty reduction strategies.

2.7 Developing an Interdependent Relationship in Disability Research: The Case of Southern Africa Federation for the Disabled (SAFOD), Psychology Department at Stellenbosch University, the African Decade of Persons with Disabilities and AfriNEAD

The Southern Africa Federation of the Disabled (SAFOD) initiated a program aimed at leveraging research to influence policy and practice concerning people with disabilities in Southern Africa. To support this effort, SAFOD-commissioned AfriNEAD to conduct an audit of disability research expertise in the region. Concurrently, the Department of Psychology at Stellenbosch University and SAFOD collaborated to train approximately twenty individuals with disabilities from SAFOD-affiliated countries in research skills. These trainees, recruited by Disabled People's Organizations (DPOs) across ten SAFOD member countries, were equipped to enhance SAFOD's institutional capacity, enabling it to design, lead and implement its own research and development initiatives. These initiatives were centred on disability issues with an inclusive focus on poverty, emancipation, social exclusion and human rights.

For the audit conducted by AfriNEAD, the SRP trainees contributed to the development of the questionnaire and were tasked with contacting at least five researchers in their respective countries to complete it. They were compensated for their work. The questionnaire was initially distributed electronically to researchers known to SAFOD who had participated in or advised on the SAFOD Research Programme (SRP). These researchers either administered the questionnaire electronically or conducted face-to-face interviews, depending on the availability of respondents. A snowball sampling technique was used, where respondents provided contact details of other suitable participants. This process, which included both SAFOD-affiliated and independent researchers, yielded a total of 87 completed questionnaires. Throughout this process, the SAFOD trainees, under the supervision of Prof. Leslie Swartz of the Psychology Department, gained valuable experience in questionnaire development and research implementation. The lead researchers for the SAFOD-commissioned audit were from AfriNEAD.

While AfriNEAD was conducting the research audit, the African Decade, also commissioned by SAFOD, requested AfriNEAD to develop a research booklet to further support the trainees' research skills. This collaboration among SAFOD, the Psychology Department at Stellenbosch, AfriNEAD and the African Decade resulted in several significant outcomes:

1. Involvement of SRP trainees in implementing research.
2. A finalized audit report of disability researchers from SADAC region.
3. A research booklet for persons with disabilities who want to be involved in research.

2.7.1 Lessons Learnt from Partnerships and Collaboration in Disability Research

This case study offers valuable insights for AfriNEAD, particularly in recognizing that persons with disabilities can play a pivotal role in shaping the research agenda. This was exemplified by SAFOD's initiative in commissioning AfriNEAD researchers to conduct a research audit for the SADC countries. Furthermore, the importance of partnerships was underscored when AfriNEAD collaborated with SAFOD research trainees—trained by the Department of Psychology—to assist in data collection. This collaboration not only provided the trainees with practical research experience but also highlighted the significance of interdisciplinary cooperation. Additionally, this period allowed the Decade to identify critical gaps and the necessity for developing a research resource booklet. Ultimately, these partnerships were mutually beneficial for all parties involved.

2.8 Chapter Conclusion

From its inception, AfriNEAD set an ambitious agenda to establish an inclusive network that leverages the skills, expertise and goodwill of researchers and disability activists. Central to this vision was the inclusion of persons with disabilities as key drivers of the network. Their resilience and networking capabilities had already led to significant achievements in advancing disability issues, particularly in framing them as matters of human rights and development. These early successes underscored the sophisticated networking skills of persons with disabilities and their critical role in disability advocacy. The chapter emphasizes the importance of partnerships in disability research, particularly the need for persons with disabilities to lead in sharing their lived experiences. The chapter concludes with a case study that further illustrates the necessity of such partnerships in advancing disability research.

References

AfriNEAD conference report. (2011). www.SUN/AfriNEAD. Stellenbosch University, Stellenbosch South Africa.

Botha, M., & Ohajunwa, C. (2024). Seeing the human behind the research: Strengthening emerging African disability researchers. *African Journal of Disability, 13*, Article a1494.https://doi.org/10.4102/ajod.v13i0.1494

Barnes, D.(2008). Exploratory talks for learning.*Research Gate*.https://doi.org/10.4135/9781446279526

Carmichael, A.(2004). The social model, the emancipatory paradigm and user involvement. In C. Barnes & G. Mercer (Eds.), *Implementing the social model of disability: Theory and research* (pp. 191–207). The Disability Press.

Chalklen, S., Seutloadi, K., & Sadek, S. (2009). *Literature review*, Southern African Federation of the Disabled, Bulawayo.

Charlton, J. I. (1998). *Nothing about us without us: Disability oppression and empowerment*. University of California Press.

Garbutt, R., & Seymour, J. (1998). '"Do we all get a PhD?" Attempting emancipatory research relating to disability in an academic environment', paper presented at the British Sociological Association Conference, Edinburgh, viewed 05 July 2013, from http://disability-studies.leeds.ac.uk/files/library/garbutt-Do-we-all-get-a-PhD-2-.pdf

Grue, J. (2011). Discourse analysis and disability: Some topics and issues. *Discourse & Society, 22*, 532–546. https://doi.org/10.1177/0957926511405572

Howell, C., Chalklen, S., & Alberts, T. (2006). A history of disability rights in South Africa. In B. Watermeyer, L. Swartz, T. Lorenzo & M. Priestley (Eds.), *Disability and Social Change South African Agenda*. HSRC.

Kachaje, R., Dube, K., MacLachlan, M., & Mji, G. (2014). The African network for evidence-to-action on disability: A role player in the realisation of the UNCRPD in Africa. *AJOD, 3*(2).

McKenzie, J., Mji, G., & Gcaza, S. (2014). With or without us? An audit of disability research in the southern African region. *AJOD*; 3 (2).

Mji, G., MacLachlan, M., Melling-Williams, N., & Gcaza, S. (2009a). Realising the rights of disabled people in Africa: An introduction to the special issue. *Disability and Rehabilitation, 31*(1), 1–6.

Mji, G., Gcaza, S., Melling–Williams, N., & MacLachlan, M. (2009b). Networking in disability for development: Introducing the African Network for Evidence-to- Action on Disability. In M. MacLachlan & L. Swartz L (Eds.), *Disability, and international development towards inclusive global health*. Springer; pp. 69–89.

Ned, L. Y., Dube, K., & Swartz, L. (2022). Challenges and opportunities of centring the African voice in disability research. *African Journal of Disability, 11*, Article a1089. https://doi.org/10.4102/ajod.v11i0.1089

Panda, S. (2024). *Leaving No One behind: Achieving the Sustainable Development Goals through Accessibility for People with Disabilities International Journal of Educational Communications and Technology (IJECT), 4*(1), 16–26.

Philpott, S., & Sait, W. (2009). An emergency submerged. In Mark Priestly (Ed.), *Disability and the life course. Global perspectives*, pp.151–166. Cambridge University Press.

Phiri, A. M. (2014). Building communities of trust: Challenges for disability. *African Journal of Disability, 3*(2), Art. #77, 3 pages. https://doi.org/10.4102/ajod.v3i2.77

Priestley, M., Waddington, L., & Bessozi, C. (2010). Towards an agenda for disability research in Europe: Learning from disabled people's organisations. *Disability & Society, 25*, 731–746. https://doi.org/10.1080/09687599.2010.505749

United Nations. (2006). Convention on the rights of persons with disabilities. Retrieved 7 August, 2023, from https://www.ohchr.org/en/instruments-mechanisms/instruments/convention-rights-persons-disabilities

World Health Organization (WHO). (2002). *Towards a common language for functioning, disability and health ICF*. World Health Organization.

World Health Organization (WHO). (2011). *World report on disability*. World Health Organization & World Bank.

CHAPTER 3

The African Network for Evidence-to-Action in Disability (AfriNEAD): A Role Player in the Realization of the UNCRPD in Africa

Gubela Mji

3.1 Introduction

The CRPD was passed by the General Assembly of the United Nations in December 2006. By February 2013, it had been signed by 155 countries and ratified by 127. It sets out key rights that citizens with a disability should enjoy in a fair society and is one of the nine core human rights treaties of the UN. The overall purpose, stated in Article 1 of the CRPD, is to "promote, protect and ensure the full and equal enjoyment of all human rights and fundamental freedoms by all persons with disabilities, and to promote respect for their inherent dignity". The elimination of discrimination by ensuring that rights may be enjoyed on an equal basis with others is a fundamental aim. While, arguably, most of the rights in the CRPD are already protected by other UN treaties, the

G. Mji (✉)
Cape Town, South Africa
e-mail: gumji@sun.ac.za

G. Mji (ed.), *Doing Disability Research in Africa*,
https://doi.org/10.1007/978-3-031-98549-2_3

CRPD frames rights in a way that is specific for persons with disabilities, a group of persons rarely referred to in those other treaties (Bartlett, 2012; Lawson, 2006). Noteworthy was the formal, active involvement of persons with Disabilities and their organizations, in the drafting and negotiations behind the development of the CRPD.

'Disability' is not formally defined in the CRPD, allowing individual State Parties considerable latitude in how they define disability in their domestic law. Persons with disabilities are characterized as follows: *persons with disabilities include those who have long-term physical, mental, intellectual, or sensory impairments which in interaction with various barriers may hinder their full and effective participation in society on an equal basis with others (UN,* 2006*)*. The use of the word 'include' in the statement above allows for a non-exhaustive description of 'Disability' that is not settled. This 'unsettledness' might be linked to the aspirations that countries might someday unanimously agree to letting go of such terms such as disability when describing part of the human family and that changing the environment we live in to an equitable structure might be part of the unifier for our humanity.

The CRPD contains the classic array of civil and political rights, such as the right to liberty (Article 14) and integrity of the person (Article 17), rights to freedom of expression (Article 21) and privacy (Article 22), the right to freedom from torture and inhumane treatment (Article 15) and rights to equal recognition before the law (Article 12) and access to justice (Article 13). It also includes economic, social and cultural rights that have come to prominence since the Second World War, including the right to home and family life (Article 23), the right to education (Article 24), and rights to health (Article 25), habitation and rehabilitation (Article 26). Some of these rights have been framed so as to have particular relevance to persons with disabilities: the right to non-discrimination (Article 5), the right to independent living and community inclusion (Article 19), the right to personal mobility (Article 20), the right to work and employment (Article 27), the right to participation in cultural life (Article 30) and the right to be free from exploitation and abuse (Article 16).

Countries are placed under a variety of obligations to take measures to modify or abolish existing discriminatory laws, regulations and practices, as well as to provide programmes to support the rights of persons with disabilities (Article 4). These obligations include, for example, a duty to provide appropriate training regarding disability issues to those involved in the administration of justice (Article 13), concrete programmes to assist people with disabilities and their caregivers to recognize and combat exploitation (Article 16), obligations to provide community support services (Article 19), and overarching duties on states to raise awareness of disability issues (Article 8) and to combat discrimination (Article 5).

The Convention further pays particular attention to the link between poverty and disability recognizing the number of Persons with Disabilities that resides in middle- and low-income countries and pledging the cooperation of the international community to assist in the realization of the Convention—it is the first international human rights treaty to have a stand-alone article—article 32—addressing International Cooperation for support of persons with disabilities in countries that are still struggling in this regard—article 32 states that:

> States Parties recognize the importance of international cooperation and its promotion, in support of national efforts for the realization of the purpose and objectives of the present Convention and will undertake appropriate and effective measures in this regard, between and among States and, as appropriate, in partnership with relevant international and regional organizations and civil society, in particular organizations of persons with disabilities (UN, 2006; Speech by previous President of Ireland, Honourable Mary Robinson, AfriNEAD conference 2007).

3.2 CRPD and MDGs in Advancement of Disability Research

The convention encourages State Parties to collect appropriate information, including statistical and research data, to enable them to formulate and implement policies to give effect to the present convention. It further expands that State Parties need to comply with internationally accepted norms to protect human rights and fundamental freedoms and ethical principles in the collection and use of research. The information collected require to be disaggregated, as appropriate, and used to help assess the implementation of State Parties' obligations under the present convention and to identify and address the barriers faced by Persons with Disabilities in exercising their rights.

Article 15 of the Convention, challenges medical and scientific experimentation without consent, and articles 5 and 16–17 prohibit research practices that are discriminatory, exploitative or violate the integrity of research participants. The precise scope of this protection will remain unclear until there is agreement, in the CRPD over what constitutes valid consent, and who can provide it. What is more, the CRPD arguably grants a right for persons with disabilities to participate in research.

There is an obligation on State Parties to support persons with disabilities involve in research and a duty to ensure that prospective research participants with disabilities have access to adequate decision-making support. In addition, the right to legal capacity gives persons with disabilities the right to decide whether to participate in research, should an opportunity present itself. Finally, the prohibition of discrimination embedded in the Convention outlaws research protocols that exclude persons with disabilities unless such exclusion can be justified and the necessary justification requires careful consideration of several interests and considerations, all of which need to be balanced.

Like the CRPD, the 2030 Agenda for Sustainable Development and its 17 Sustainable Development Goals (SDGs) pledge to leave no one behind and recognize disability as an issue that cuts across all SDGs. The adoption of SDGs by the United Nations in 2015 provide a blueprint for achieving a better and more sustainable future for all (United Nations, 2015). However, despite the SDGs' ambition to leave no one behind, persons with disabilities are often overlooked in the global development agenda. This implies that there is more that need to be done.

Ghai (2009) located disability issues within the discourse of the Millennium Development Goals (MDGs), highlighted the reasons for the absence of persons with disabilities from the MDGs agenda and called for the expansion of democratic space to ensure that their rights were given due consideration. The identification of accessible resources that have contributed to the achievement of the SDGs for persons with disabilities indicates the need for increased investment, collaboration and awareness to ensure that no one is left behind in the pursuit of sustainable development. The relationship between disability and specific SDGs, including SDG 4, SDG 8, SDG 10, SDG 11 and SDG 17, demonstrates how achieving these goals can positively impact persons with disabilities and the world.

3.3 Previous Perspectives Underlying Disability Research Practice

For the past decade, disability researchers have been involved in a debate about how disability research should be framed and conducted. This debate has centred on ideology (the uses and intent of research), research ethics and methodology. The wider disabled population holds many of the arguments forwarded by critics of traditional disability research. Perhaps given that 'scientific' research has perpetuated, reproduced and legitimated the marginalization of persons with disabilities, justifying segregation, eugenics and the denial of civil rights, it should be of little wonder that disabled people are suspicious of disability research, especially by non-disabled researchers (Mji et al., 2009a, b; Phiri, 2014; Rioux & Bach, 1994).

Disability research has been viewed as mostly one-sided and dominated by a group of mainly British sociologists. It has been argued that traditional research on disability issues is flawed and problematic in several respects (Barnes, 1992; Oliver, 1992; Stone & Priestley, 1995; Zarb, 1992). Most crucially, these commentators have argued persuasively that disability research is not representative of disabled peoples' experiences and knowledge. This, they contend, is because disability discourse has been—and to a large degree still is—overwhelmingly dominated by people who are not disabled, and most of the research is conducted by non-disabled researchers. They argue that it is only persons with disabilities who can know what it is like to be disabled and so it is only persons with disabilities who can truly interpret and present data from other persons with disabilities. Moreover, they note that research concerning disability research is invariably researcher-orientated, based around the desires and agendas of the (non-disabled) researcher and able-bodied funding agencies rather than subject(s) of the research (persons with disabilities).

In other words, existing research has largely been a source of exploitation rather than liberation (Barnes & Mercer, 1997). Drawing on work within feminism, they argue that power-relations within the research process need to be destabilized, and the research agenda wrestled free from academic researchers still using traditional research methodologies. As such, they called for the adoption of research strategies that are both emancipatory (seeking 'positive' societal change) and empowering (seeking 'positive' individual change through participation).

Since the disability movement in Africa used literature mainly drawn from the North regarding their arguments, it appeared that when AfriNEAD presented its 1st AfriNEAD conference in 2007, these were some of the main concerns that emerged from the disability movement. Many African disability researchers did not contribute to disability research at that time.

3.4 African Response to Disability Research

Comaroffs (2011) in Swartz (2014) argues that the days when scholars and researchers in the Global South would be consumers and adapters of theory and expertise from the North are over: indeed, if the North wants to address its own emergent issues, the people to learn from may well be researchers embedded in Global South contexts, as they seem to come with practical solutions that are facing disability research. We may not yet be at a stage where we can claim that disability research in sub-Saharan Africa has come of age, but it is probably fair to say that we are in a process of maturing and starting to be seen as growing up. With this increasing maturity, and substantially increasing visibility, comes a growing responsibility (Swartz, 2014). Swartz (2014) further expands that this is an exciting and challenging time for disability research in the region, some of the challenges are related to experience, expertise, enumeration, evidence and expectations. There are also theoretical concerns as most of disability theories and arguments have been coined in the North (Phiri, 2014; Nguyeni, 2018; Ohajunwa et al., 2022; Dwadwa-Henda, 2023). In this regard I want to share the case of the late Mr Alexander Phiri the previous Chairperson of SAFOD on his thinking about disability research in Africa (Table 3.1).

Disability studies in the African region is an emerging scholarship. Previously most disability theories that guide the development of educational programs and scope of practice in Africa, emerge from the Global North (Dwadwa-Henda, 2023; Mji & Ohajunwa, 2021; Nguyeni, 2018). The lens used for the exploration of disability, as a concept, and the lived experiences of persons with disabilities, have predominantly emanated from the Global North until now, when disability academic scholars from the South are emerging (Mji & Edusei, 2019). These understandings of disability from the Global North are constructed through social processes and philosophical influences that inform and position groups within society, instituting a hierarchy of people and groups. This includes

Table 3.1 Owning the African research agenda

Owning the African research agenda: Late Mwanza Alexander Phiri African Journal of Disability (AJOT) 2014
Unfortunately, the distinction between developed and developing societies, for example, is often that of one group of researchers or academics dominating the other (MacLachlan et al., 2010). I hate racism because it should not have any space in this modern world; but the issue of race is critical in their search agenda in Africa and there is a need to address this issue. Africa faces the greatest challenge of establishing and making use of its own research for effective decision-making in development programmes and policymaking. However, our budgets for research and development are not sufficient and can be augmented by those of our colleagues in developed countries. Also, our own governments are not as committed as those in developed countries claim to be to evidence-based actions. We therefore require research staff from developed countries to support the development of the research evidence which is critical for effective policy development and implementation in our countries
Our research budgets in Africa should be increased so that we generate our own data to back up our campaigns for meaningful development. We Africans have for too long relied on external researchers, on externally generated data and externally driven research agendas that do not effectively address our issues. If we do not own the research, how can we address our needs? African people must invest in home-grown research capacity and research solutions that will meet the specific needs of Africa. This, however, does not mean that we are saying 'no' to international partnerships. Yes, we want to work with our international partners, but they should allow us to drive the research agenda. Our partnership should be genuine and based on the principle of equality
Dr Sindiso Ngwenya (2009), Secretary General of the Common Market for Eastern and Southern Africa (COMESA), maintains that there is a need for Africans to collect their own data to tell the African story, and to benchmark themselves against development targets. Ngwenya warns that if we do not collect our own data, we will make plans using the wrong data. I agree with him. We need to promote a kind of research which is useful; research that solves daily problems and makes a positive impact on people's lives, rather than research that is merely for academic purposes. We should not look only at researchers in universities in developed countries as the traditional research community, but also at the emerging research tools and initiatives in developing countries that are embedded in the rich, strong African culture, as being equally authentic for the work at hand

conceptualization of disability within societies which has been influenced by identity politics and historical foundations (Mpofu & Harley, 2006).

Bezzina (2018) points to the role of indigenous knowledge in the understanding and development of interventions for and with persons with disabilities. Ned, Kpobi and Ohajunwa (2022) further support this thinking in their paper on thinking about mental health and spirituality from the Indigenous knowledge systems frame of reference. African researchers and persons with disabilities need to lead the dialogue on

African theories on disability in the Global South (Chimbala-Kalenga, 2015; Kolawole, 2005). Ohajunwa (2019), Setume (2016) highlighted how the Global South conceptualizes disability from a metaphysical-spiritual location of disability, using a more collectivist approach. Africans' belief system is underpinned by inclusive relationships (Mji, 2012; Ohajunwa, 2019). In many cultures, the perception and description they have towards a person with impairment and disability is that of a person struggling with some form of functionality, which to them is not a unique thing as from time-to-time some family members do struggle from functionality problems (Mji, 2012; Dwadwa-Henda, 2023).

While African researchers can be critical of research and theories coming from the Global North, they also need to avoid approaching disability research as if they are starting from a blank slate; instead, they must use a critical lens that will question and replace what is not relevant for countries with appropriate research evidence (Mji & Ohajunwa, 2021; Nguyeni, 2018). Drawing a leaf from an indigenous scholar Tinky-Penny who suggested a backward and forward movement when addressing issues of decolonization. He recommended a critical examination of information from the North before using it in the South, whereby there might be a need to connect and understand how that aspect is addressed in the South and check whether it seems better than the aspect from the North. This will determine what should be used for the future in the Global South and what should be left behind, thereby preventing the proverbial 'throwing the baby with the bath water' (Tinky-Penny in Mji, 2012).

Persons with disabilities in Africa are not yet experiencing meaningful change in their quality of life, access to equal rights and a level of community integration, despite a favourable policy environment in some countries and a supportive research evidence base. Real change and social development are still required to realize a truly inclusive society (Mji et al., 2009a). Inclusive policies that facilitate all people to access equal human rights will assist in unlocking the potential of people with disabilities to make contributions to the development agenda in their various countries. The African Network for Evidence-to-Action in Disability (AfriNEAD) was established in response to the challenges highlighted above and the historical context of exclusion and exploitation in disability research. It aims to address the gaps identified by promoting inclusive approaches and fostering dialogue among African researchers and persons with disabilities.

The vision of the African Network for Evidence-to-Action on Disability (AfriNEAD) is premised on the need to use existing and new knowledge and evidence from a diverse range of research topics and sources. AfriNEAD facilitates a multidimensional, intersectoral, interactive forum that focuses on how the evidence that is generated by disability researchers is translated to action (Mji et al., 2011). AfriNEAD also affords disability researchers exposure to the complexities of the issues of equity within the disability field and the need to see disability as a social and developmental issue. AfriNEAD is a forum that builds and sustains relationships, partnerships and cooperation between researchers and users of research evidence and knowledge. The forum provides a platform where research results are better able to target and influence policy and practice—AfriNEAD lives in the research-policy-practice 'gaps' seen as 'problems' in other fora. Realizing that such 'problems' present the greatest opportunities for learning and enacting learning is the driving force behind AfriNEAD (Mji et al., 2011). In the next session I will present how AfriNEAD had contributed to the implementation of the CRPD.

3.5 AfriNEAD a Role Player in Implementation of CRPD

Recently, disability researchers argued that involving persons with disabilities in disability discourse as controllers or partners offers practical and social gains for persons with disabilities. In line with the thinking of young persons with disabilities as asserted in a paper by Rule and Modipa (2012) stating, "We must believe in ourselves" and they seem to think that this belief in themselves will assist them to become the drivers of their own programs. It is only with their active involvement that disability discussions will reflect their needs, concerns and interests (Heap et al., 2009; Tilley et al., 2021). Through their participation and partnership, research will become more reflexive, reciprocal and representative (McKenzie et al., 2014; Goldberg & Kleintjes, 2022). It will provide a platform from which persons with disabilities (PWDs) can speak for themselves, seek services and support what they want, explicitly influence social policy and advocate for disability rights (Tilley et al., 2021).

In short, research will become enabling and empowering. Inclusion acknowledges and signifies respect for the valuable and worthwhile contributions of disabled co-researchers (Rohleder et al., 2021). Here the co-researcher's expertise is acknowledged as equal but from a different frame of reference than the academic. Capitalizing then on the combined impetus afforded by the *African Decade for Persons with Disabilities (1999)* and the *United Nations Convention on Rights for Disabled People (CRPD) (2006)* the focus of AfriNEAD was on how to combine research, policy and practice to realize the rights of persons with disabilities in the African region (Mji et al., 2009a, b).

The CRPD was adopted in December 2006 and ratified with unprecedented support from states, including those on the African continent. The CRPD aims to *promote, protect and ensure* the full and equal enjoyment of all human rights and fundamental freedoms by all persons with disabilities, and to promote respect for their inherent dignity (CRPD, 2006). In a large measure the development of the CRPD was precipitated by the remarkable work of disabled peoples' organisations (DPOs) who contributed to the development of white papers in their own countries such as South African Integrated National Disability Strategy White Paper of 1997. These documents are usually preceded, guided and supported by constitutional imperatives of those countries that developed the documents (*Constitution of the Republic of South Africa, 1996)*. However, CRPD ratification is only the first step in a long process that African states parties must undertake to manifest and provide needs that will impact positively in the lived experiences of persons with disabilities (Strnadová, 2022). It is in this regard that AfriNEAD took an inclusive human rights-based approach to research ensuring that research produced by AfriNEAD is aligned with the CRPD (Kachaje et al., 2014; Mji et al., 2009a, b).

Some of the important events conducted by AfriNEAD are the tri-annual regional conferences. In 2009 AfriNEAD started to present its conference in eight thematic areas that were developed from compressing the 50 articles of the CRPD (AfriNEAD conference report, 2009). These nine thematic areas are:

- Children & Youth with Disabilities,
- Education: Early Childhood to Tertiary,
- Economic Empowerment,
- Development Process in Africa: Poverty, Politics and Indigenous Knowledge systems,
- Health and HIV & AIDS,
- Community-Based Rehabilitation,
- Holistic Wellness: Sport, Recreation, Sexuality and Spirituality,
- Research evidence (Kachaje et al., 2014),

- Assistive Technology (later integrated in 2020).

When an AfriNEAD conference is announced, researchers are invited to present abstracts that fit in these eight thematic areas. AfriNEAD further capitalizes on the CRPD Implementation Toolkit, under the theme, *The ABC of Research Evidence-to-Action: putting CRPD principles into action for rights-based change (CRPD, 2006)* (Kachaje et al., 2014).

Hence researchers are asked to examine their work and present papers in the eight thematic areas, demonstrating how the evidence-to-action concept could be put into practice; and to plan how AfriNEAD could be operationalized within the CRPD ABC framework that is:

A: Adopt a rights-based vision
B: Build a constituency for change
C: Counting successes and setbacks.

The ABC of Research Evidence-to-Action: putting CRPD principles into action for rights-based change chimes closely with the 2030 Sustainable Development Goals (SDGs) agenda (Panda, 2024). In the same spirit as the CRPD, SDGs commits to empower those at risk of vulnerability, including persons with disabilities. The SDGs also promotes universal respect for human rights, equality and non-discrimination with inclusion of persons with disabilities at its heart requesting and committing not to leave anyone behind and to reach the furthest behind first. Since the SDGs goals and targets are based on equality and non-discrimination, **no** goal can be achieved if a part of the population, such persons with disabilities, are forgotten (Panda, 2024). It is in this regard that researchers are asked to take note of the following when preparing papers for the AfriNEAD conference/s (Table 3.2).

The end-product of presentations in each thematic area is a set of resolutions that can be used to highlight the specific disability-related issues to key stakeholders in each field. The conference research outcomes for that conference that are summarized from the eight thematic areas are consolidated into a special issue published by the African Journal of Disability (Kachaje et al., 2014).

It is important to mention that in disability research, some practitioners overtly avoided ethical requirements because of their resource implications. When these principles are inadequately addressed, the resulting research is of reduced quality and can damage trust in the research

Table 3.2 Aspects to consider for papers for AfriNEAD conferences

1. What constitutes good research evidence?
2. What evidence already exists?
3. What evidence is still needed? (Where are the gaps in Africa and internationally?)
4. How do we facilitate evidence-based research?
5. How do we facilitate evidence-to-action in this area?
6. How can we include the following areas in research and evidence-based practice development?
    - Human rights for people with disabilities
    - Accountability: of the rights-holders (the people claiming their rights) and the duty-holders (the people who have the duty to protect and promote enjoyment of the rights in question)
    - Empowerment of rights-holders
    - Full participation of all relevant stakeholders
    - Non-discrimination and attention to vulnerable groups—specific attention to issues like discrimination, equality, equity and groups of persons who have been particularly marginalized
7. What practical steps can we take to keep connected within AfriNEAD to build and maintain momentum in this area?

process among persons with disabilities. Persons with disabilities expressed concerns about the lack of inclusion during the research process and the oversight of certain ethical principles required for conducting research, especially in disability research (Barnes, 2008; Tilley et al., 2021).

There is a danger that poor-quality research conducted without careful attention to ethical practice might lead to a poor knowledge base underpinning changes in policy and service provision for persons with disabilities. Hence from the inception of AfriNEAD, we aimed to encourage the use of emancipatory ethical research methodologies among the network researchers (Kachaje et al., 2014; Mji et al., 2009a, b; Strnadová et al., 2022). Emancipatory research is based on a social model of disability, which engages persons with disabilities in all stages of the research process, and has a transformative aim, aiming to improve the lives of persons with disabilities (Barnes, 2008).

3.5.1 *Challenges and Opportunities for AfriNEAD in Using a Right-Based Instrument Such as the CRPD in Disability Research in Africa*

As explained under 3.4, in 2009 AfriNEAD decided to use the Convention on the Rights of Persons with Disabilities (CRPD) as an instrument that guides AfriNEAD disability research. AfriNEAD took the fifty articles of the CRPD and compressed them into eight thematic areas (which later were revised to nine thematic areas due to the addition of the thematic area on assistive devices) (Ebuenyi et al., 2023) to drive the AfriNEAD research evidence (Kachaje et al., 2014). The CRPD is an heir of the UN Standard Rules on the Equalization of Opportunities for Persons with Disabilities, adopted in 1993 (Sait, 2023). The CRPD is a human right-based instrument that aims to *promote, protect and ensure* the full and equal enjoyment of all human rights and fundamental freedoms by all persons with disabilities, and to promote respect for their inherent dignity (Sait, 2023; Kahonde & Mji, 2024). Using a human right-based instrument such as the CRPD offers both challenges and opportunities for AfriNEAD and disability research in Africa.

According to de Man (2018), a human rights approach contribute[s] to a holistic approach to eradicating poverty and promoting development. The human rights approach also focuses on holding governments and other actors accountable for their actions, and by so doing promotes a more efficient use of resources (by promoting access to information and fighting corruption). de Man (2018) further expands that the purpose of human rights is to avert, as far as possible, the social conditions and practices that history teaches us which, inevitably lead to human suffering and misery. de Man (2018) further warns that though human rights approaches appear to have positive outcomes, human rights practitioners must take note of critiques and challenges and be willing to adapt existing practices and theories to address criticisms.

Some of the challenges linked to a human rights instrument such as the CRPD in the African region are terms such as development. Cornwall and Eade (2010) in their book on: Deconstructing Development Discourse challenges the authenticity of such term. They further expand that 'development' has been used by donors for the so-called development programs in the areas classified as third worlds. When you try obtaining specifics and accountability for this term, you discover that this is a term happily said by donors in the knowledge that it will have no significant consequences and accountable to the constituents they are addressing (Cornwall & Eade, 2010). Indigenous People of African descent especial those residing in rural areas and who a majority still aligns themselves to indigenous practises are used to being classified as undeveloped or underdeveloped. These groups of people have experienced the looking down upon their knowledge systems by modernity. Hence the term development within the African region might be questioned about whose development, by whom and what requires to be developed (Mji, 2019).

Human rights that are strongly embedded in the CRPD raises another controversy when it comes to individual rights versus collective rights. According to some critics, there is an inherent incompatibility between individual human rights and collective rights, both from a legal and from an ideological perspective. For some human rights are only individual rights and cannot include group rights (Kanade, 2022). Lately individual rights have been heavily supported by development programs geared towards improving the lives of persons with disabilities (Dwadwahenda, 2023). Trying to gain access to these programs that focus on individual rights has the potential to alienate persons with disabilities from their families and communities, especially those living in indigenous rural communities. Mji and Ohajunwa (2021) points to the fact that Indigenous communities tend to lean more on collective rights that are underpinned by Ubuntu. They further expand that using Ubuntu on Indigenous rural communities has the capacity to support a contextually and culturally relevant reconceptualization of disability. Disability is a social construct, hence disability and the several ways that persons with disabilities are supported in rural areas should be understood and informed by the prevailing social context of these indigenous spaces.

The use of CRPD as an instrument that drives AfriNEAD research focus area must be applauded. Much as there is criticism about rights that are enshrined within the CRPD, for AfriNEAD this opens an opportunity to further work on domesticating and decolonizing the CRPD. The AfriNEAD network has opened opportunities about dialogue on disability research by developing a network with an inclusive group of stake holders (Disabled people, academics, business, government and civil society). Domestication of the CRPD depends on the collective thought and dialogue of these stakeholders. Mladenov (2013) points to how the CRPD quickly gained the number of signatories on the first day of the CRPD's opening for signature in the UN. Mladenov (2013) further reminds us that the consensus over the CRPD is built upon decades of sustained activism on behalf of disabled people's organizations. Persons with disabilities are experienced in resolving challenging problems using the collective approach (Mji & Ohajunwa, 2021).

The model built by AfriNEAD of disability research country working groups (DRCWGs) discussed in Chapter 7 of this book offers opportunities for domestication and decolonizing the CRPD. The DRCWGs are mini AfriNEAD embedded within countries affiliated with AfriNEAD. They too use the nine thematic areas used by AfriNEAD that emerged from the CRPD and the same design as AfriNEAD for AfriNEAD stakeholders participating in these countries. Mji and Ohajunwa (2021) maintains that understanding of lived experience of disability is expressed differently within various African Indigenous communities. It is hoped that DRCWGs can be able to offer this disability experience through exploration of the nine thematic areas developed from the CRPD. Central to the AfriNEAD stakeholders participating in these countries are persons with disabilities embedded within their countries and within the DRCWGs. The core argument is that persons with disabilities as a collective should be recognized and admitted as important stakeholders and contributors in the community that interprets and gives the CRPD its African meaning (Mji and Ohajunwa, 2021). It is argued that persons with disabilities civic self-organizing is indispensable for sustaining the interpretation of the CRPD along transformative and emancipatory lines (Mladenov, 2013). AfriNEAD with its nine thematic areas developed from the CRPD offers opportunities for the domestication and decolonizing the CRPD.

3.6 Chapter Conclusion

To end this chapter, it is important to mention that Article 31 of the CRPD emphasize that the research evidence-to-action approach should ensure that research benefits make a difference to the lives of persons with disabilities. AfriNEAD was initiated with the intention of improving relationship between persons with disabilities and researchers (Kachaje et al., 2014; Mji et al., 2009a, b). This response involved the creation of a flat platform for persons with disabilities, disability researchers, Government representatives, Civil Society Formations and business to dialogue how disability research evidence can be used as a prong for the realization of persons with disabilities in the African Region. Central to this dialogue are persons with disabilities with AfriNEAD responding to the adjunct that says: “nothing about us without us” (McKenzie et al., 2014). The research evidence-to-action approach should ensure that research benefits make a positive difference to the lives of persons with disabilities. Regarding AfriNEAD’s intention to disability research, the CRPD is rightfully positioned to drive the development of the research themes for AfriNEAD. AfriNEAD with its DRCWGs offers possibilities for the domestication of the CRPD and decolonizing disability research.

References

AfriNEAD Conference reports. (2007, 2009, 2011, 2014, 2017, 2020 & 2023).

Bach, K. (1994, June). Conversational implicature, mind and language, Vol. 9, No. 2. https://doi.org/10.1111/j.1468-0017.1994.tb00220.x

Barnes, C. (2008). An ethical agenda in disability research: Rhetoric or reality? In D. M. Mertens & P. E. Ginsberg (Eds.), *The handbook of social research ethics* (pp. 458–473). Sage.

Barnes, C. (1992). Qualitative research: Valuable or irrelevant? *Disability, Handicap and Society, 7*, 139–155.

Barnes, C., & Mercer, G. (Eds.). (1997). *Doing disability research*. University of Leeds, Disability Press.

Bartlett, M. (2012). Going (Digitally) native. *Journal of Animation, 7*(3). https://doi.org/10.1177/1746847712459597

Bezzina, L. (2018). The role of indigenous and external knowledge in development interventions with disabled people in Burkina Faso: the implications of engaging with lived experiences. *Disability and the Global South, 5*(2), 1488–1507. https://www.researchgate.net/publication/327012134

Botha, M., & Ohajunwa, C. (2024). Seeing the human behind the research: Strengthening emerging African disability researchers. *African Journal of Disability, 13*, Article a1494. https://doi.org/10.4102/ajod.v13i0.1494

Chimbala-Kalenga, R. (2015). Adjusting western research techniques to accommodate research in the indigenous realm. *Indilinga: African Journal of Indigenous Knowledge Systems, 14*(1).

Comaroff, J., & Comaroff, J. L. (2011). Theory from the south: Or, how Euro-America is evolving toward Africa. *Anthropological Forum, 22*(2), 113–131. https://doi.org/10.1080/00664677.2012.694169

Cornwall, A., & Eade, D. (2010). Deconstructing development discourse: Buzzwords and Fuzzwords. Practical Action Publishing Ltd. Warwickshire, CV23 9QZ, UK. www.practicalactionpublishing.org

de Man, A. (2018). Critiques of the human rights framework as the foundation of a human rights-based approach to development. *Journal for Juridical Science, 43*(1), 84–116. https://doi.org/10.18820/24150517/JJS43.v1.5

Dwadwa-Henda, N. (2023). *Experiences of persons with disabilities of Xhosa rituals and traditions, which contribute to health and wellbeing*. Stellenbosch University.

Ebuenyi, I. D., Smith, E. M., Jamali, M. Z., Munthali, A., & MacLachlan, M. (2023). The IDEAL PROCESS for developing assistive technology policy.

Assistive Technology, 36(3), 224–231. https://doi.org/10.1080/10400435.2023.2254359

Ghai, A. (2009). Disability and the millennium development goals. *Journal of Health Management, 11*(2), 279–295. https://doi.org/10.1177/097206340901100202

Heap, M. Lorenzo, T., & Thomas, J. (2009). We've moved away from disability as a health issue, it's a human rights issue': reflecting on 10 years of the right to equality in South Africa. *Journal Disability & Societ, 24*(7), 857–868.

Kachaje, R., Dube, K., MacLachlan, M., & Mji, G. (2014). The African network for evidence-to-action on disability: A role player in the realisation of the UNCRPD in Africa. *AJOD, 3*(2).

Kahonde, C. K., & Mji, G. (2024). Disability research in African Network for evidence-to-Action in disability affiliated countries. *AJOD, 13*, 1–9, 2226–7220. (online). https://doi.org/10.4012/ajod.v13i.1517

Kanade, M. (2022). Foundations of international human rights law IV: Collective rights.

Kolawole, D. (2005). Concepts of politics. In D. Kolawole (Ed.), *Readings in political science* (pp. 1–14). Dakaal Publishers.

Lawson, B. (2006). How designers think: The design process demystified (4th ed.). Elsevier/Architectural Press.

MacLachlan, M., Carr, S. C., & McAuliffe, E. (2010). *The aid triangle: Recognizing the human dynamics of dominance, justice and identity.* Fernwood Publishing.

McKenzie, J., Mji, G., & Gcaza, S. (2014). With or without us? An audit of disability research in the southern African region. *AJOD*, 3(2).

Mji, G. (2013). *The health knowledge utilised by rural older Xhosa women in the management of health problems in their home situation, with a special focus on indigenous knowledge [Doctoral Thesis].* University of Stellenbosch.

Mji, G., MacLachlan, M., Melling-Williams, N., & Gcaza, S. (2009a). Realising the rights of disabled people in Africa: An introduction to the special issue. *Disability and Rehabilitation, 31*(1), 1–6.

Mji, G., Gcaza, S., Melling–Williams, N., & MacLachlan, M. (2009b). Networking in disability for development: Introducing the African network for evidence-to-action on disability. In M. MacLachlan & L. Swartz (Eds.), *Disability, and international development towards inclusive global health.* Springer, pp. 69–89.

Mji, G., Gcaza, S., Swartz, L., MacLachlan, M., & Hutton, B. (2011). An African way of networking around disability. *Disability and Society; 26*(3).

Mji, G., & Edusei, A. (2019). An introduction to a special issue on the role of assistive technology in social inclusion of persons with disabilities in Africa: Outcome of the fifth African network for evidence-to-action in disability conference Afr. *J Disability*. https://doi.org/10.4102/AJOD.v8i0.681

Mji, G., & Ohajunwa, C. (2021). *Ubuntu ethics and human rights: Implications for rehabilitation practices in indigenous African families of persons with disabilities (PWDs).* Midrand KR Publishing.

Mladenov, T. (2013). The UN convention on the rights of persons with disabilities and its interpretation. *Alter: European Journal of Disability Research, 7*(1), 69–82. https://doi.org/10.1016/j.alter.2012.08.010

Mpofu, E., & Harley, D. A. (2006). Racial and disability identity: Implications for the career counselling of African Americans with disabilities rehabilitation. *Counseling Bulletin, 50*(1), 14–23. https://doi.org/10.1177/00343552060500010301

Ned, L., Kpobi, L., & Ohajunwa, C. (2022). Thinking about mental health and spirituality from the Indigenous knowledge systems frame of reference. *Disability Studies Quarterly, 41*(4). https://doi.org/10.18061/dsq.v41i4.8450

Nguyeni, X. T. (2018). Critical disability studies at the edge of global development: Why do we need to engage with Southern theory? *Canadian Journal of Disability Studies, 7*(1), 1–25. https://doi.org/10.15353/cjds.v7i1.400

Ngwenya, S. N. (2019). COMESA of the common market for the eastern Nand Southern Africa. *Published by the Order of the Council of Authority*

Panda, S. (2024). *Leaving No One behind: Achieving the Sustainable Development Goals through Accessibility for People with Disabilities International Journal of Educational Communications and Technology (IJECT), 4*(1), 16–26.

Phiri, A. M. (2014). Building communities of trust: Challenges for disability. *African Journal of Disability, 3*(2), Art. #77, 3. https://doi.org/10.4102/ajod.v3i2.77

Priestley, M., Waddington, L., & Bessozi, C. (2010). Towards an agenda for disability research in Europe: Learning from disabled people's organisations. *Disability & Society, 25*, 731–746. https://doi.org/10.1080/09687599.2010.505749

Ohajunwa, C. O. (2019). *Understanding, interpretation and expression of spirituality and its influence on care and wellbeing: An explorative case study of a South African Indigenous community.* Stellenbosch University.

Ohajunwa, C. O., Mji, G., & Chimbala-Kalenga, R. (2022). Encouraging reciprocal healthcare practice within a South African Indigenous community. *AlterNative: An International Journal of Indigenous Peoples, 18*(1), 141–146. https://doi.org/10.1177/11771801221085631

Oliver, M. (1992). Changing the social relations of research production. *Disability, Handicap and Society, 7*, 101–114.

O'Cinneide, C. (2009). Extracting protection for the rights of persons with disabilities from human rights frameworks: Established limits and new possibilities. In O. M. Arnardóttir & G. Quinn (Eds.), *The UN Convention on the Rights of Persons with Disabilities: European and Scandinavian Perspectives* (pp. 163–198). Martinus Nijhoff Publishers.

Rioux, M. H., & Bach, M. (1994). *Disability is not Measles*. Canadian cataloguing in publication data.

Robinson, M. (2007). Speech at the First AfriNEAD conference (SSEAD). Stellenbosch South Africa.

Rohleder, P., Braathen, S. H., Chiwaula, M., Hunt, X., & Swartz, L. (2021). Creative collaboration on disability and sexuality action research project. A reflective diary account. *Qualitative Research in Psychology, 18*(2), 250–270. https://doi.org/10.1080/14780887.20181499837

Rule, P., & Modipa, T. R. (2012). "We must believe in ourselves" attitudes and experiences of adult learners with disabilities in KwaZulu-Natal, South Africa. *Adult Education Quarterly, 62*(2), 38–158.

Sait, W. (2023). An exploration of disability experiences and responses of disabled persons and their families within Muslim culture of the community of Strand, South Africa. PhD thesis. Stellenbosch University, South Africa.

Setume, S. D. (2016). Myths and beliefs about disabilities: Implications for educators and counsellors, pp. 62–76 | Published online: Download citation https://doi.org/10.1080/23312521.2016.1152938

South African Constitution. (1996). Republic of South Africa, South Africa.

South African Integrated National Disability Strategy White Paper. (1997). Retrieved 7 August, 2023, from http://www.info.gov.za/whitepapers/1997/disability.htm

Stone, E., & Priestley, M. (1995). 'Parasites, pawns, and partners: Disability research and the role of non-disabled researchers. *British Journal of Sociology, 47*, 696–716.

Strnadová, I., Dowse, L., & Garcia-Lee, B. (2022). *Doing research inclusively: Co-production inaction*, Disability Innovation Institute, UNSW, Sydney.

Swartz, L. (2014). Five challenges for disability-related research in sub-Saharan Africa. *African Journal of Disability, 3*(2), 149.

Tilley, E., Strnadová, I., Ledger, S., Walmsley, J., Loblinzk, J., Christian, P. A., et al. (2021). "Working together is like a partnership of entangled knowledge" Exploring the sensitivities of doing participatory data analysis with people with learning disabilities. *International Journal of Social Research Methodology, 24*(5), 567–579. https://doi.org/10.1080/13645579.2020.1857970

Tinky -Penny Indigenous scholar in Mji, G. (2013). *Exploring the health knowledge carried by older Xhosa women in their home situation, with special focus on Indigenous knowledge* [Stellenbosch]. https://scholar.sun.ac.za/items/4c2431c5-5387-4697-a626-8d8a781b4c3f

United Nations. (2006). *Convention on the rights of persons with disabilities*. Retrieved 7 August, 2023, from https://www.ohchr.org/en/instruments-mechanisms/instruments/convention-rights-persons-disabilities

Zarb, G. (1992). On the road to Damascus: First steps towards changing the relations of disability research production. *Disability, Handicap & Society, 7*(2), 125–138. https://doi.org/10.1080/02674649266780161

CHAPTER 4

AfriNEAD Considerations and Response in Conducting Ethical-Driven Disability Research

Gubela Mji

4.1 Introduction

Article 31 of the UNCRPD emphasizes that research evidence-to-action approach should ensure that research makes a difference and benefits the lives of persons with disabilities. AfriNEAD has been concerned with the relationship between persons with disabilities and disability researchers. Persons with disabilities had questioned the lack of inclusion during the process of research, the overlooking of some ethical principles required in conducting research and how persons with disabilities are presented in disability research (Mji et al., 2013). As stated in Chapter 3 under Sect. 3.4, authors such Kachaje et al. (2014) and Strnadová et al. (2022) argue that there is a danger that poor-quality research without careful

G. Mji (✉)
Cape Town, South Africa
e-mail: gumji@sun.ac.za

G. Mji (ed.), *Doing Disability Research in Africa*,
https://doi.org/10.1007/978-3-031-98549-2_4

attention to ethical practice might result in poor information that influence the changes required in policy and service provision for persons with disabilities.

Oliver (1992) points to the fact that previous research methodologies were inconsiderate to persons with disabilities as they alienate, disempower and disenfranchise disabled research participants. People with disabilities, due to power imbalances, place their knowledge into the hands of the researcher to interpret and make recommendations on their behalf while they do not have a clue about the resources that are available to ensure that such recommendations can come to fruition, because the researchers are not part of the communities where persons with disabilities reside. Additionally, some of these recommendations might not be a priority for persons with disabilities in that context. Barnes and Mercer (1997) and Kitchin (2005) are concerned about existing research which they see has largely been a source of exploitation rather than liberation for persons with disabilities. They further expand that persons with disabilities are calling for the adoption of research strategies that are both emancipatory (seeking 'positive' societal change) and empowering (seeking 'positive' individual change through participation). Getting close to this inspiration by Barnes and Mercer (1997) and Kitchin (2005) would require research practices that are underpinned by good ethical practice.

One of the greatest intentions of disability research, as one of the instruments for realization of rights of persons with disabilities, is to ensure that it remains responsive to its constituency (Oliver, 2022). Approaches and methodologies that follow narrow visions need to be challenged and research evidence must include plans which consider resources needed for implementation (Balton, 2022). Often different groups of researchers repeat the same research questions to the same people with disabilities as they overlook the critical stage of developing research protocols that include their participants during the development stage (Dwadwa-Henda, 2023).

AfriNEAD was developed and implemented against this backdrop. There was a need to improve relationships and bridge the gap between disability researchers and persons with disabilities who usually act as participants in disability research (Mji et al., 2009). By developing the DABGC Consortium that links disability, academia, business, government and civil society, AfriNEAD had an ambition that the divide, created by how disability research is operationalized by academic researchers, can be revisited and improved. AfriNEAD wanted to be an inclusive network drawing on the best skills, expertise and goodwill of researchers and disability activists. There was a desire for a mutual exchange of skills, knowledge and resources within the DABGC Consortium. This might have appeared as an ambitious goal, but the network was focused into the future and intends to level out the playing field in disability research by creating opportunities within the network whereby persons with disabilities will enjoy equal opportunities. Disability researchers needed to constantly examine their scope of practice, to ensure they were underpinned by research ethics (Mji et al., 2013). The next section provides the background to this chapter.

4.2 Background

When AfriNEAD was established in 2007, it developed a diverse "community of practice" to provide evidence and ways of using this evidence to improve the lives of persons with disabilities in Africa (Mji et al., 2009). It was to be an inclusive network drawing on the best skills, expertise and goodwill of researchers and disability activists. The goal was to bring together a broad community of stakeholders that could bridge the divide between persons with disabilities and researchers. This divide between persons with disabilities and research practitioners was clearly visible at the 2007 and 2009 conferences. In the third AfriNEAD conference in Zimbabwe in 2011 with the title, Building Communities of Trust, AfriNEAD wanted to directly address and bridge this divide between disability researchers and persons with disabilities. At the centre of this divide was how persons with disabilities view disability researchers regarding disability research, as they felt that the way disability research was conducted was unethical.

Considering past human rights abuses and exploitative practices in research with vulnerable groups, it is important to develop specific ethical benchmarks to empower vulnerable groups, such as persons with disabilities, to question, guide and control the nature and process of research about themselves (Mji et al., 2013). For persons with disabilities, Part of this control included persons with disabilities participating in planning, execution and interpreting aspects of disability-related research (not just being participants/subjects). Disability researchers in AfriNEAD were aware of the marginalization of persons with disabilities within the region, hence it was important to consider the politics of relationships as disability researchers, and how these impact on the participants themselves. Critical research debates were happening in AfriNEAD with the goal of ensuring that research is conducted in an ethical manner. There was a need to be explicit about the role researchers play to avoid the misconception that research can provide resources for persons with disabilities (Nama & Swartz, 2002). NDA (2024) warns that in the past, society, by its actions and omissions, had sometimes worsened the position of persons with disabilities. Disability activists such as Alexandria Phiri (2014) frown at practices such as euthanasia and tend to see these approaches as inhuman.

In Africa, there is also a challenge that many persons with disabilities remain encased in households that practice and are guided by indigenous principles. Disability researchers conducting research tend to use ethical approaches and theories based on the Global North. Sefotho (2021) explains that indigenous ontologies have for many centuries endured epistemological subjugation from Euro-Western epistemologies. Widdows (2011) points to the need to understand and respond to, the impact of colonialism and its history within contemporary bioethics with special focus on covert, rather than overt, conversion of others to one's own values by presentation of these values as universal and requiring acceptance. Doing disability research in households that practice indigenous knowledge systems, one might need to explore ethics and human rights as influenced by the lens of Ubuntu. Ubuntu as an indigenous ethic has the capacity to support a contextually and culturally relevant reconceptualization of disability research. Ubuntu as a moral ethic for disability research, when engaging with persons with disabilities and their families will have a far-reaching effect (Mji & Ohajunwa, 2021). The area of ethics in disability research continued to be a focus area for disability practitioners that are affiliated with AfriNEAD. The next section present ethics considerations in conducting disability research in AfriNEAD.

4.3 Ethics Considerations in Conducting Disability Research in AfriNEAD

Disability research ethics are located within the wider research ethics frameworks. Ethics principles require that any research involving human subjects is framed and conducted in a way that respects the human rights and dignity of the individuals concerned (Bryen, 2016a, b). In what was previously classified as advancing scientific knowledge through human experimentation, persons with disabilities and other vulnerable groups were used as convenient research participants (Bryen, 2016a, b). Although society has moved from this blatant misuse of vulnerable groups, including persons with disabilities, there is still concern by persons with disabilities about whether they will not be harmed, are safe and represented in an acceptable manner (McDonald et al., 2015).

AfriNEAD aimed to develop a flat platform that envisaged inclusion, appropriate representation and equal participation of persons with disabilities (Kahonde & Mji, 2024). This in disability research brought a new thinking about disability and vulnerability in disability research (Iacono & Carling-Jenkins, 2012; Dwadwa-Henda, 2025). There was a need to transform disability research with persons with disabilities playing different roles (participating, conducting, commissioning and disseminating) (Iacono & Carling-Jenkins, 2012; Mckenzie et al., 2014). Such thinking chimes closely with what persons with disabilities have been saying about their abilities and disabilities for a long time (Rule & Modipa, 2012). AfriNEAD have chosen the UNCRPD as a guide for practitioners in conducting disability research. Article 31 of the UNCRPD gives clarity to areas that matter most to persons with disabilities (UNCRPD, 2006). The UNCRPD guiding principles in conducting disability matters put emphasis on understanding that human rights are about respect for the inherent dignity and including the freedom to make one's own choice in matters that concern persons with disabilities (NDA, 2024). Disability researchers and Practitioners within AfriNEAD have seen these guiding principles as an inspiration and a goal to strive for. Some of these principles are contained in article 31 of the UNCRPD. Below in Table 3.1 is the presentation of principles of article 31 (Table 4.1).

Table 4.1 outlines the principles of article 31 of the UNCRPD. These principles relate to matters that are about working with persons with disabilities. They also relate to disability research and researchers. There is a need to unpack what each principle means in doing research with persons with disabilities, taking into consideration the need for fluid approaches and context. In the previous chapter AfriNEAD compressed the 50 articles of the UNCRPD to ensure the relevancy of disability research within AfriNEAD. On matters of ethics in disability research it stands to reason for AfriNEAD affiliated researchers to draw guidance from the UNCRPD. Other guidelines that are also relevant and important to research and also relate to disability research are included in ethics and research protocols of human research committees of different institutions. Section 4 below present two case studies to show how AfriNEAD

Table 4.1 Article 31 of the UNCRPD

Article 31 of the UNCRPD The principles of the present Convention: • Respect for inherent dignity, individual autonomy including the freedom to make one's own choices, and independence of persons; • Non-discrimination; • Full and effective participation and inclusion in society; • Respect for difference and acceptance of persons with disabilities as part of human diversity and humanity; • Equality of opportunity; • Accessibility; • Equality between men and women; • Respect for the evolving capacities of children with disabilities and respect for the right of children with disabilities to preserve their identities

affiliated disability researchers and practitioners responded and considered ethical disability research matters when doing disability research.

4.4 Presentation of Two Case Studies That Demonstrate Response and Considerations by AfriNEAD-Affiliated Researchers in conducting Disability research

Ongoing dialogue and debates in AfriNEAD-assisted AfriNEAD-affiliated researchers to develop an awareness and sensitivity towards issues of human rights and dignity of persons with disabilities and other vulnerable groups when doing research. Below in the presentation of two case studies that demonstrate on how this response and consideration was outplaying at practical level when doing disability research. These case studies are as follows:

a. Development of ethics guidelines for taking photographs of vulnerable populations.
b. Assistive technology information mapping project (AT-Info-Map).

4.4.1 *Development of Ethics Guidelines for Taking Photographs of Vulnerable Populations*

It has become a common practice for many researchers and human rights activists to use photographs as a way of drawing attention to the public plight of those at the margins who might at that time be experiencing some form of vulnerability (Mji et al., 2013). Mji et al., (2013) further highlight how the use of images in research lacks a history of accepted ethical practice or a range of theoretical positions on which researchers can base ethical judgements. The issue of proper representation of persons with disabilities using photographs is always problematic. At the same time, however, one of the keyways in which disability has been managed and stigmatized, has not been through problematic display but rather by concealment and the removal of people with disabilities from the mainstream (Mji et al., 2013). This has been done both by confining people with disabilities to institutions far away from the public gaze, and by the systematic silencing of disability issues and people with disabilities from the media in general. Garland-Thomson (2009) in Mji et al., 2013, encourages disability researchers to avoid histories of exclusion and hiding, and instead to present the lives of persons with disabilities in an empathetic rather than in an othering and stigmatizing manner. The case study below demonstrates how AfriNEAD partnered with the Human Research Ethics Committee (HREC) of Stellenbosch University, South Africa, in developing guidelines for taking photographs in vulnerable populations (Table 4.2).

4.4.2 *Assistive Technology Information Mapping Project (AT-Info-Map)*

The issue of assistive technology (AT) is seen as a fundamental need for persons with disabilities to access other rights and needs, like health, education, employment, independent living and social participation. It is a challenge to envisage full inclusion and participation of persons with disabilities without appropriate AT. In sub-Saharan African countries and other low- and middle-income countries (LMICs), there are minimal to non-existent accurate statistical estimates on the availability of ATs for Persons with Disabilities. In LMICs, the provision of assistive products is inadequate, with poorly structured systems in place to improve and facilitate service delivery (Borg et al., 2011; Visagie et al., 2019). One

Table 4.2 Case study 1—Developing guidelines for taking photographs for vulnerable populations

We were part of a group of researchers affiliated with AfriNEAD and investigating issues of access to health services for persons with disabilities in four countries in Africa. The South African-based group collected data in rural, urban and peri-urban areas spread across three provinces. At the start of data collection, we had no plan or clear protocol for taking photographs. This raised the question of what a responsible approach to taking photographs should be within the context of research. Given the negative historical use of photographs of people with disabilities, as described above, we wanted to consider whether there are other, more positive, potential uses of visual images. We started with the rural site and after the first research visit, we presented our problem of lacking guidelines to the Human Research and Ethics Committee (HREC) of Stellenbosch University with the intention of obtaining guidelines from the Department for taking photographs. The response we got was that there were no guidelines and that the Department would be interested in developing such guidelines with the researchers. Before we started developing these guidelines with the HREC Department, we went back to the rural area, as in this area we were able to observe a lot of marginalization and vulnerabilities experienced by the community, including persons with disabilities. We wanted to hear from persons with disabilities their views on both the potential negative effects and benefits of taking photographs of persons with disabilities. We conducted a small qualitative study using face-to-face interviews with six participants who were persons with disabilities. A summary of the findings from this study pointed to the fact that persons with disabilities welcome being photographed and put in the local newspaper as this might improve their visibility and enhance their dignity, especially if they are photographed performing some of the activities that persons without disabilities perform. This would further remove assumptions about their disabilities and highlight their abilities. What was clear in their minds was that they object to photographs being taken of them without their consent, and three of the participants said that they would consider legal action in such a situation. Participants did not wish to be party to a situation in which their images benefited others at their own expense (Mji et al., 2013). Equipped with this information from this small qualitative study conducted amongst persons with disabilities in the remote rural area of South Africa—we felt this information coincided with literature on taking photographs amongst persons with disabilities and other vulnerable groups of people. We were able to go back to the HREC Department to start developing guidelines for taking photographs with vulnerable groups (attached in appendix one is the HREC guidelines for researchers and research ethics committee prepared by Gubela Mji and Nicola Barsdorf in 2013).

of the biggest challenges for persons with disabilities is to locate where they could find providers for AT. Faced with this challenge of where to locate AT, Southern Africa Federation for Disabled (SAFOD) based in Gaborone in Botswana, together with AfriNEAD at Stellenbosch University in South Africa, Washington, University in Seattle, America; and Dimagi in Cape Town, South Africa, championed Assistive Technology

Information Mapping Project (AT-Info-Map) in 2016. This project was funded by the Google Impact Challenge as one of the *'big ideas that will use technology to expand opportunity and independence for people with disabilities'*. At that time AfriNEAD was involved in the Global Cooperation on Assistive Technology (GATE) which is a World Health Organization (WHO) initiative, drawing together people who share the GATE vision: a world where assistive technology (AT) is universally accessible to everyone, everywhere. The WHO aimed to get governments of all countries affiliated with the WHO to ensure that ATs are accessible and affordable to persons with disabilities in their countries. Below is the case study on assistive technology information mapping project (AT-Info-Map) (Table 4.3).

Table 4.3 Case study 2—Assistive Technology Information Mapping Project (AT-Info-Map)

When Google made a call for projects that address the *'big ideas that will use technology to expand opportunity and independence for people with disabilities'*, Google wanted applicants from the NGO sector
As a response to the Google call, AfriNEAD approached SAFOD who at that time, had the affiliation of ten Southern African countries. In a dialogue with the Chairperson of SAFOD, the perception was that our response should link with the GATE project. The Chairperson of SAFOD came with the idea that although AT is a challenge for persons with disabilities, the greatest challenge was how to locate the scarce AT providers. SAFOD then suggested that the theme of the project should be how technology can be used as a vehicle to supply information on how to easily gain access to AT, hence the INFO-MAP project. AfriNEAD then further linked with Washington University in Seattle in the USA, who were AT specialists, and they further linked with Dimagi, a technical specialist who will use their technology system (Comcare) to create a customized App that collects and provides information about AT availability in Southern Africa for mapping support. The SAFOD-led INFO-MAP project that started in 2016 lasted for three years
The project outcomes were: (1) developing a Portuguese version of the app; (2) testing with Talk Back, a built-in screen reader on Android phones, to ensure data entry and data searching were accessible to persons with visual impairments; (3) reducing data demand of the app; and (4) creating training resources such as manuals and online videos to assist app access and usage, and educate the general public about AT (Visagie et al., 2019)
During its tenure, the SAFOD-led project was able to liaise with the GATE project in the WHO. The project participants presented their research findings at the 2017 AfriNEAD Ghana conference with its theme: Disability and inclusion in Africa: the role of assistive devices. An article was published by the African Journal of Disability regarding this project (Visagie et al., 2019)

4.4.3 *Discussion of the Two-Case Study*

The first case study presents the contesting issue of using photographs with vulnerable groups, including persons with disabilities (Mji et al., 2013). Photographs in journals, textbooks and conference presentations are sometimes included to draw attention and catch the eye of readers (Mji et al., 2013). They also add value in medical education by enhancing the text using pictorial examples. The person in the photograph is, however, often seen as an interesting case or finding, rather than a living, feeling person. Images of vulnerable groups of people, such as people struggling from HIV and AIDs, indigenous people and disabled people, are often used as a tool to highlight some of the challenges they are experiencing (Mji et al., 2013). Botha and Ohajunwa (2024) frown upon research that overlooks the human behind the research. When AfriNEAD affiliated researchers noted the omission of guidelines in taking photographs while doing research by their Human Research Ethics Committee (HREC) department, they were accountable and took it upon themselves to ensure that HREC of Stellenbosch University was made aware of this paucity. Not only did they report this challenge but were also willing to join hands with HREC in developing these guidelines, thereby demonstrating their accountability to both persons with disability and the academic institution (Barnes, 2003).

The mini qualitative research study they developed before the start of developing these guidelines was in line with the adjunct of "nothing about us without us" (Charlton, 1998; Mji et al., 2013). These researchers did not want to discuss these guidelines without first speaking to persons with disabilities about their views on both the potential benefits and negative effects of taking photographs of persons with disabilities. Persons with disabilities from the rural area wanted their photographs taken and put in a local newspaper as this would assist with the need for advocacy and improve their visibility in the rural area where the small qualitative study was done. Using the same notion of "nothing about us without us", what these persons with disabilities were clear about was that their photographs should not be taken without their consent (Mji et al., 2013). The need for their consultation was paramount to them as this gives them control of the images that were about them. Booth et al. (2003) and Boxall et al. (2009) encourage first consulting with persons with disabilities about the images they want to be taken and if possible, give the camera to them to take the images, thereby giving them full control. The mini qualitative research study assisted the AfriNEAD researchers to work with the HREC committee using information from this rural research site that was informed by this small group of persons with disabilities.

The second case study highlighted the importance of involving persons with disabilities in various roles in disability research. What is important to persons with disabilities is for persons with disabilities and their organizations to be sometimes involved in setting the research agenda as well as conducting, commissioning and disseminating the research (Mckenzie et al., 2014). Google was rightful in requiring responses for its funding call for a project that involved persons with disabilities not to come from academic institutions but from within the Non-Governmental Organization (NGO) as abilities and disabilities are commonly ascertained at this level and this where the greatest need for financial support is needed. For AfriNEAD it was again an opportunity to work with a partner that is an organization for persons with disabilities. In this project persons with disabilities could set the research agenda (Barnes, 2008; Kitchin, 2005). SAFOD was rightfully suitable to lead the Assistive Technology Information Mapping Project (AT-Info-Map) as SAFOD had the following assets for the research: 10 SAFOD-affiliated countries (Botswana, Zambia, Namibia, Zimbabwe, Lesotho, Swaziland, Mozambique, Angola, Malawi and South Africa), the national DPOs in the SAFOD-affiliated countries, AT providers, local organizations that serve persons with disabilities and knowledge about government officials within these countries (Visagie et al., 2019). Persons with disabilities are clear in their thinking that they have both abilities and disabilities—what they need are equal opportunities to participate (Rule & Modipa, 2012). Persons with disabilities are concerned about the misinterpretation of their needs (Charlton, 1998). They argue that they have both the experience of being disabled and know what their needs are. Regarding accessing AT by persons with disabilities in the ten SAFOD countries, the SAFOD Chairperson knew what the main problem was and how to design the aim for the Google research project.

4.4.4 Chapter Conclusion

There exists a history of exclusion and oppression of PWDs in Africa that results in mistrust and suspicion from many disability activists. The whole research enterprise creates tensions and an atmosphere of hostility between disability activists and disability researcher practitioners (Balton, 2022). At the core of these tensions was the lack of inclusion of persons with disabilities in research. Mistrust and hostilities were also experienced during the hosting of the first and second AfriNEAD conferences in 2007 and 2009. The third AfriNEAD conference with the title: Building Communities of Trust: Evidence-to-Action in Disability Research conference in 2011, aimed to address some of these tensions. The dialogue in AfriNEAD conferences afforded space for these tensions to be addressed. Persons with disabilities find it unethical to only be participants in disability research as they see themselves as having the skills to act in different roles in disability research. Some of the debates which related to matters of inclusion and representation in disability research were already happening in AfriNEAD since its inauguration in 2007. These debates were starting to create an awareness on disability research practitioners affiliated to AfriNEAD. These researchers did not only see inclusion of persons with disabilities in disability research as ethical, but also as beneficial, as shown in the Info-Map Project. This also give an opportunity to raise awareness on ethical concern/s in academic Departments such as the HREC Department of Stellenbosch University as it has been shown by the issue of absence of guidelines for taking photographs in vulnerable populations. Both researchers and persons with disabilities benefit from using ethical compassionate approaches in disability research.

References

Balton, S., Arvidsson, P., Granlund, M., Huus, K., & Dada, S., (2022). Test-retest reliability of picture My participation in children with intellectual disability in South Africa. *Scandinavian Journal of occupational Therapy, 29*(4), 315–324. 10.1080/11038128.2020.1856922

Barnes, C. (2003). What a difference a decade makes: Reflections on doing 'emancipatory' disability research. *Disability & Society, 18*(1), 3–17. https://doi.org/10.1080/713662197

Barnes, C. (2008). An ethical agenda in disability research: Rhetoric or reality? In D. M. Mertens & P. E. Ginsberg (Eds.), *The handbook of social research ethics* (pp. 458–473). Sage.

Barnes, C., & Mercer, G. (1997). Breaking the mould: An introduction to doing disability research. In C. Barnes & G. Mercer (Eds.), *Doing Disability Research.* The Disability Press.

Booth, T., & Booth, W. (2003). In the frame: Photovoice and mothers with learning difficulties. *Disability & Society, 18*(4), 431–442.

Borg, J., Larson, S., & Ostergren, P. O. (2011). The right to assistive technology: For whom, for what and by whom. *Disability & Society*, *26*(2), 151–167.

Botha, M., & Ohajunwa, C. (2024). Seeing the human behind the research: Strengthening emerging African disability researchers. *African Journal of Disability, 13*, Article a1494. https://doi.org/10.4102/ajod.v13i0.1494

Boxall, K., & Ralph, S. (2009). Research ethics and the use of visual images in research with people with intellectual disability. *Journal of Intellectual and Developmental Disability, 34*(1), 45–54.

Bryen, D. N. (2016). Ethical issues in conducting research involving persons with disability: A view from the past and some new challenges. *Humanities and Social Sciences, 4*(53). https://doi.org/10.11648/j.hss.s.2016040201.18

Bryen, D. A. (2016). Ethical Issues in conducting research involving persons with disability: A view from the past and some new challenges. *Humanities and Social Sciences. Special Ethical Sensitivity: A Multidisciplinary Approach*, 4(2–1), 53–59. https://doi.org/10.11648/j.hss.s.2016040201.18

Charlton, J. I. (1998). *Nothing about us without us: Disability oppression and empowerment*. University of California Press.

Dwadwa-Henda, N. (2023). *"Experiences of persons with disabilities of Xhosa rituals and traditions, which contribute to health and wellbeing", PhD thesis* (Issue March) [Open Access, Stellenbosch University]. https://scholar.sun.ac.za/handle/10019.1/128429

Geiger, M., Luger, R., Mckenzie, J., & Morris. S. (2019). Collaborative development of a draft code of ethics for research with persons with disabilities in Cape Town Selected References. Conference: Public Health Association of South Africa (PHASA), Cape Town South Africa.

Jenkins, S. (2012). Editorial. *International Journal of Sports Science and Coaching, 7*(4), III - IV. ISSN 1747–9541https://doi.org/10.1260/1747-9541.7.4

Iacono, T., & Carling-Jenkins, R. (2012). The human rights context for ethical requirements for involving people with intellectual disability in medical research. *Journal of Intellectual Disability Research., 56*, 1122–1132. https://doi.org/10.1111/j.1365-2788.2012.01617.x.[DOI][PubMed][GoogleScholar]

Kachaje, R., Dube, K., MacLachlan, M., & Mji, G. (2014). The African network for evidence-to-action on disability: A role player in the realisation of the UNCRPD in Africa. *AJOD, 3*(2).

Kahonde, C. K., & Mji, G. (2024). Disability research in African network for evidence-to-action in disability affiliated countries. *African Journal of Disability, 13*, Article a1517. https://doi.org/10.4102/ajod.v13i0.1517

Kitchin, R. (2005). *Towards emancipatory and empowering disability research: Reflections on three participatory action research projects*. National University of Ireland Maynooth.

McDonald, K. E., Schwartz, N. M., Gibbons, C. M., & Olick, R. S. (2015, April). "You can't be cold and scientific": community views on ethical issues in intellectual disability research. *J Empir Res Hum Res Ethics, 10*(2), 196–208. https://doi.org/10.1177/1556264615575512. Epub 2015 Mar 13. PMID: 25769310; PMCID: PMC4399491

McKenzie, J., Mji, G., & Gcaza, S. (2014). With or without us? An audit of disability research in the southern African region. *AJOD*, 3(2).

Mercer, C. (1997). *Students with learning disabilities (5th.ed).* New jersey. Prentice – hall. Inc.

Mji, G., MacLachlan, M., Melling-Williams, N., & Gcaza, S. (2009). Realising the rights of disabled people in Africa: An introduction to the special issue. *Disability and Rehabilitation, 31*(1), 1–6.

Mji, G., & Ohajunwa, C. (2021). *Ubuntu ethics and human rights: Implications for rehabilitation practices in indigenous African families of persons with disabilities (PWDs).* Midrand KR Publishing.

Mji, G., & Edusei, A. (2019). *An Introduction to a Special Issue on the Role of Assistive Technology in Social Inclusion of Persons with Disabilities in Africa: Outcome of the Fifth African Network for Evidence-to-Action in Disability Conference Afr J Disabil.* https://doi.org/10.4102/ajod.v8i0.681

Mji, G., Schneider, M., Vergunst, R., & Swartz, L. (2013). On the ethics of being photographed in research in rural South Africa: Views of people with disabilities. *Disability & Society.* https://doi.org/10.1080/09687599.2013.84410

Nama, N., & Swartz, L. (2002). Ethical and social dilemmas in community based controlled trials in situations of poverty: A view from a South African project. *Journal of Community and Applied Social Psychology, 12*, 286–297.

NDA (National Disability Authority). (2024). Ethical Guidance for Research with Disabled People, Dublin, Ireland.

Oliver, M. B. (2022). Social media use and eudaimonic well-being. *Current Opinion in Psychology, 45,* Article 101307. https://doi.org/10.1016/j.copsyc.2022.101307

Oliver, M. (1992). Changing the social relations of research production. *Disability, Handicap and Society, 7*, 101–114.

Phiri, A. M. (2014). Building communities of trust: Challenges for disability. *African Journal of Disability, 3*(2), Art. #77, 3. https://doi.org/10.4102/ajod.v3i2.77

Rule, P., & Modipa, T. R. (2012). "We must believe in ourselves" attitudes and experiences of adult learners with disabilities in KwaZulu-Natal, South Africa. *Adult Education Quarterly, 62*(2), 38–158.

Sefotho, M. M. (2021). Basotho ontology of disability: An Afrocentric onto-epistemology. *Heliyon, 7*(3), 8. https://doi.org/10.1016/j.heliyon.2021.e06540

Strnadová, I., Dowse, L., & Garcia-Lee, B. (2022). *Doing research inclusively: Co-production inaction*, Disability Innovation Institute, UNSW, Sydney.

United Nations. (2006). *Convention on the rights of persons with disabilities*. Retrieved 7 August, 2023, from https://www.ohchr.org/en/instruments-mechanisms/instruments/convention-rights-persons-disabilities

Visagie, S., Matter, R., Kayange, G., Chiwaula, M., Harniss, M., & Kahonde, C. (2019). Perspectives on a mobile application that maps assistive technology resources in Africa. *African Journal of Disability, 8*, Article a567. https://doi.org/10.4102/ajod.v8i0.567

Widdows, H. (2011). Western and eastern principles and globalized bioethics. *Asian Bioethics Review, 3*(1), 14–22.

CHAPTER 5

AfriNEAD Conferences

Gubela Mji, Callista Kahonde, Marcia Lyner-Cleopha, Anthony Edusei, Allister Munthali, and Hillary Lane

5.1 Introduction

There has been a general perception that networks can substantially scale up the effectiveness of the existing resources and achieve equitable distribution of such resources (Daar et al., 2007; De Bont et al., 2007; Lau, 2004; Mozunder & Marathe, 2007). Friedman et al. (2007) suggest that the network aspect of social capital is also useful to best understand the active, on-the-ground processes by which people of some countries, beset with poverty, racial/ethnic subordination and internal divisions (arising from inequalities at different levels) and other marginalized groups, such as persons with disabilities, defend their own and other peoples' rights and dignity through networking. One of AfriNEAD's objectives and an

G. Mji (✉) · C. Kahonde · M. Lyner-Cleopha · A. Edusei · A. Munthali · H. Lane
Cape Town, South Africa
e-mail: gumji@sun.ac.za

C. Kahonde
e-mail: ckkahonde@sun.ac.za

M. Lyner-Cleopha
e-mail: cleophas@sun.ac.za

G. Mji (ed.), *Doing Disability Research in Africa*,
https://doi.org/10.1007/978-3-031-98549-2_5

important tool for networking is the hosting of triennial Africa-wide conferences focusing on a particular issue of interest to assess progress on evidence-to-action and showcase action to evidence and to consolidate and take the debate forward.

When members of a network congregate in an AfriNEAD conference, around a specific concept, they are not starting from a point of knowing, but from a cup that is not yet full, and the degrees of not being full vary from member to member. There are also other spaces of the network regarding concepts about which the members might lack knowledge. The starting point is to accept this fact and not be threatened by it. The use of dialogue and debate assist in the osmosis of ideas, including the germination and sprouting of completely new ideas. This suggests that the network is suspended in its planning and development through a process-orientated ideology that is driven and facilitated by communication.

For networks to function and move forward there should be clear communication and minimal neutrality regarding the core goal of the network. This communication approach is integral for bridging the gap between philosophy and concept to action. The strength of being able to play out this function of bridging up the gap between philosophy and concept to action is related to the ability of the network to allow multiple, conflicting ideas to evolve. By allowing these conflicting ideologies, lessons and learning to evolve, we move away from the thinking that we live in a world that says you are either with us—which implies you are our friend—or against us implying that you are our enemy. Within AfriNEAD, there was an approach to guard against a tendency towards 'group thinking' and the AfriNEAD conferences were a platform to unite diverse opinions to ensure that different approaches and solutions are used to address the marginalization of persons with disabilities in Africa.

A. Edusei
e-mail: eduseiak@gmail.com

A. Munthali
e-mail: amunthali@palmconsulting.mw

H. Lane
e-mail: hillarylane@outlook.com

Since its inauguration in 2007, AfriNEAD intended to host two conferences in South Africa consecutively and subsequently, three further conferences to be held consecutively in other African countries. After three conferences hosted in other African countries outside South Africa, two AfriNEAD conferences will again be hosted in South Africa. By hosting the AfriNEAD conferences in other African countries, the goal was to learn from these countries about the status of disability issues in their countries, to encourage accessibility of the environment like hotels where the conference is being held and to network closely about disability issues with key stakeholders such as government departments in the country. The rationale for hosting two consecutive conferences in South Africa was to ensure that AfriNEAD gets an opportunity to strengthen the AfriNEAD Secretariat and support Stellenbosch University, Stellenbosch, South Africa, on its journey of being an inclusive University by using the conference as a platform. The first two international conferences (2007 & 2009) were in Cape Town, South Africa, the following three (2011, 2014 & 2017) were in Zimbabwe, Malawi and Ghana. The 2020 and 2023 conferences were again hosted in Cape Town, the 2026 conference and the two thereafter, will be hosted in other African countries. In the next section the background to this chapter is given.

5.2 Background

One of the objectives of AfriNEAD was to host triennial international conferences focusing on a particular issue of interest to network members. Initially (2007–2009) the conferences were hosted biennially as symposia and were meetings that addressed how strong research evidence can be put into advocacy, policy and rehabilitation practice, identifying facilitators and barriers, and drawing on persons with disabilities, carers, clinicians, managers, NGO's, civil servants, civil society, research funders and politicians. These symposia would invite researchers to present their work to policymakers and disability practitioners and challenge them to think-through the steps necessary to realize AfriNEAD's potential. This would produce a unique and stimulating collection of papers from each symposium that would be published as a special issue of a suitable international journal. Initially, papers from the first symposium were published in the International Journal of *Disability & Rehabilitation*. Subsequent special issues were then published in the *African Journal of Disability* (AJOD) once AfriNEAD in collaboration with Division of Disability and Rehabilitation Studies (DDRS) and Kwame Nkrumah University of Science and Technology (KNUST) in Kumasi, Ghana, established this journal. These special issues would have a distinct theme depending on the theme of the conference. Later the name symposium was changed to conference as people felt this would have a better impact when applying for funding to come to the conference. The AfriNEAD Secretariat also requested the Governing Body responsible for governance of AfriNEAD to host the conferences after every three years instead of two as more time was needed to prepare for the next conference.

The breadth of stakeholders in the domain of disability is enormous and indeed one of the functions of the network was to engage a wide array of individuals and organizations through an evidence-based dialogue. In Chapter 2, Sect. 5 in this book, the challenges related to developing trust amongst different stakeholders have already been explained. AfriNEAD needed an approach on how the network will interface and develop trusting relationships with these stakeholders. It was not only sufficient to explore how AfriNEAD may be able to support their activities, and how they can provide guidance to researchers regarding how disability research can be used as a prong to address challenges facing persons with disabilities in the region including their involvement in different areas in the research process, i.e. drivers, participants, enumerators, etc. There was also a need for a space for dialogue between persons with disabilities and researchers that would assist to build a bridge that will be a unifier between these stakeholders. The AfriNEAD conference was seen as a platform where these stakeholders could engage on equal footing to focus on how disability research evidence could realize the rights of persons with disabilities in the region.

Secondly, there was a sense that the AfriNEAD conference will not only be a platform for dialogue but also a platform to produce disability research evidence which could be harnessed into outputs such as special issues. Thirdly, there was a perception that the conference would be an information sharing platform on how scarce resources related to disability research can be identified, located and shared amongst various entities that are engaged in disability research. Fourthly, there was hope that attendees of AfriNEAD conferences from various countries would be able to meet and network on how to start developing clusters of disability researchers in their own countries of origin; to ensure that production of disability research can happen in their own countries; and for AfriNEAD to have a vehicle for dissemination of the conference resolutions. Lastly, disability studies is an emerging scholarship within the African region, most of the disability theories that guide the development of educational programmes and scope of practice in Africa, emerge from the Global North. During the conference, it was hoped that the AfriNEAD stakeholders would start to dialogue on African theories on disability and how these theories could facilitate the advancement process of realizing the rights of persons with disabilities in the region. In the next section research focus areas for AfriNEAD conferences are presented.

5.3 Research Focus Areas for the AfriNEAD Conferences—The AfriNEAD Commissions

As stated in Chapter 3 of this book, in 2009 AfriNEAD started to present its conference in thematic areas that were developed from compressing the 50 articles of the UNCRPD (AfriNEAD conference report, 2009). The rationale was to ensure that research presented in AfriNEAD conferences by researchers and practitioners was aligned with the CRPD. Initially these thematic areas were six and were:

Research evidence, CBR, HIV/AIDS, education, land rights, youth and lifestyle issues, as well as issues of indigenous knowledge systems. These thematic areas were later refined for the conference presented in 2011 as presented in Table 5.3 (Table 5.1).

These thematic areas remained the same until 2017 when the commission on assistive technology was added. The commission on research

Table 5.1 Eight (8) Thematic areas are for presentation of AfriNEAD conference since 2011

Eight (8) Thematic areas are for presentation of AfriNEAD conference since 2011
• Children & Youth with Disabilities, • Education: Early Childhood to Tertiary, • Economic Empowerment, • Development Process in Africa: Poverty, Politics and Indigenous Knowledge systems, • Health and HIV & AIDS, • Community Based Rehabilitation, • Holistic Wellness: Sport, Recreation, Sexuality and Spirituality, • Research evidence

Kachaje et al. (2014)

evidence had been moved to plenary at some of the conferences because conference attendees wanted to hear what was discussed in this area, but for the 2023 conference, researchers and disability practitioners sent abstracts that were directly linked to this commission—hence it has remained as part of the commissions. The next section presents the process of selecting a hosting country.

5.4 The Process of Selecting a Hosting Country: The Bidding Process

The AfriNEAD conference programme is usually extensive as its intention is to ensure that all voices are heard regarding how disability research evidence can be used as a prong to realize the rights of persons with disabilities in Africa. The conference usually takes three days. The last item to be addressed in the conference programme is the Annual General Meeting (AGM) which reports on items that are brought by the Governing Body of AfriNEAD to the agenda of the AGM for decision-making. All conference attendees are invited to attend the AGM, which gives the attendees an opportunity to see the governance of AfriNEAD in action. The items for discussion and approval by the AGM are critical aspects that will guide the AfriNEAD Governing Body for the next three years. As part of the agenda, there is a point for countries to bid to host the next conference. The AGM chair invites attendees from different countries to bid to host the conference. Countries that have offered to enter the conference bidding process are sent a bidding document developed by the Secretariat and asked to develop a proposal that addresses all aspects that are highlighted by the bidding document. This is to ensure that countries have considered the implications of hosting the conference. The bidding countries will be given a time by when they should return the completed bidding document. The AfriNEAD Secretariat will read the proposals from the bidding countries and will select the proposal of a country that seems better prepared to host the conference. The only time that this process has not been followed was for the hosting of the first three AfriNEAD conferences: at that time AfriNEAD was still on a learning curve on how AfriNEAD conferences should be hosted. Even when the conferences are hosted in South Africa/Stellenbosch University, the Bidding Document is still used as a guide for preparations to host the conference. In the next section, support given to a hosting country is discussed.

5.5 Support Given to a Hosting Country

The bidding process requires that the country that will host the conference to complete a bidding document that is approved by the AfriNEAD Secretariat. This document covers aspects such as: the development of the conference organizing committee; the different portfolios within the conference organizing committee that will assist in the preparation for the conference, which will include the budget committee. The conference theme and rationale for theme selection is also given in this document. The draft conference programme is given which includes suggestions for keynote speakers.

Once a country has been selected to host the conference, the AfriNEAD Secretariat will visit the hosting country twice. The first visit is aimed at meeting the conference organizing committee, visiting the conference hosting venue and checking issues of accessibility and meeting with key in-country stakeholders such as disabled people organizations (DPOs), Government officials, academics and business. The second visit is assessing the readiness of the country to host the conference and to iron out any loose ends. During the conference, the Secretariat acts as a springboard for advice and support for the hosting country. It is important that research paper presentations and discussions will ultimately be translated into conference resolutions and recommendations. The conference will end with an AGM where aspects that will guide the network for the next three years will be discussed, including the bidding process for countries who aim to host the next conference. After the conference, a conference report will be developed by the hosting country working together with the AfriNEAD Secretariat to produce a conference report. Researchers and disability practitioners that have presented papers will be encouraged to translate their papers for publications for a conference special issue to be published in the African Journal of Disability (AJOD).

5.6 Themes Related to the AfriNEAD Conferences

Each conference has had a specific theme related to where the process of engagement with AfriNEAD stakeholders was about realizing the rights of persons with disabilities in the region. When conferences were hosted by Stellenbosch University, Stellenbosch, South Africa, the theme was discussed by the Governing Body, as within this structure many countries (both African and international countries) that are affiliated to AfriNEAD are represented. Although the titles are all different and each targeting a specific focus area, they have been informed by the articles of the United Nations Convention on the Rights of Persons with Disabilities (UNCRPD) since 2009. When conferences are held by countries outside South Africa, those countries, after completing the proposal for the bidding document, also present the theme for the conference and the rationale thereof. In Sect. 5.6 the themes for the seven AfriNEAD conferences (2007–2023) and rationale for selection of each theme are listed as follows.

5.6.1 *The First Stellenbosch Symposium on Evidence-to-Action in Disability (SSEAD)*

This theme was for the first Stellenbosch symposium on evidence-to-action in disability which was hosted in 2007 in Cape Town, South Africa, and which gave birth to AfriNEAD. The conference title that included the evidence-to-action part was to assist the conference attendees to connect with the focus of AfriNEAD.

5.6.2 *The ABC of Research Evidence-to-Action: Putting UNCRPD Principles into Action for Rights-Based Change*

This was the theme for the second AfriNEAD symposium hosted in 2009 in Cape Town, South Africa. It was during the planning of this conference that AfriNEAD recognized the critical role of domesticating the UNCRPD principles in Africa. The network worked on crafting themes that capture the essence of the UNCRPD principles and used them as a framework to organize research that was presented at the conference as well as resolutions and recommendations emanating from that research. This conference had six commissions based on the six research areas derived from UNCRPD Articles. The ABC of Research Evidence-to-Action: putting UNCRPD principles into action for rights-based change was drawn from the evaluation tool of the UNCRPD which reminded presenters and conference attendees the importance of assessing one's work on how it is aligned with some of the core concepts and principles of the UNCRPD.

5.6.3 *Building Communities of Trust: Evidence-to-Action in Disability Research*

This was the theme for the third conference hosted in Zimbabwe in 2011. Upon further deliberation, the network decided to refine the themes and produced seven commissions based on the UNCRPD, that guided research presented at this conference. Now AfriNEAD had to reflect on the process of developing inclusive research communities, which was not easy as AfriNEAD was rightfully bringing people from different sectors to work together—it became clear to the network that without trust this would be an impossible task.

5.6.4 *Intensifying Disability Research and Practice to Achieve the MDGs in Africa: Our Experience and Aspirations for the Future*

This theme was for the fourth conference presented in Malawi in 2014. The theme was geared towards seeing the continuation of AfriNEAD's promotion of the UNCRPD principles on the continent by calling for research guided by the UNCRPD-informed themes. Again, upon further reflection it was decided to divide one of the commissions into two themes. Therefore, this conference attracted research that was packaged according to eight commissions informed by the UNCRPD. It was also the exciting time of the Millennium Development Goals (MDGs)—and disability advocates highlighted that persons with disabilities were left out of the MDGs. Through the advocacy of persons with disabilities and some AfriNEAD representatives, persons with disabilities were included during the development of the Sustainable Development Goals (SDGs).

5.6.5 *"Disability and Inclusion in Africa: The Role of Assistive Technology"*

This was the theme for the fifth AfriNEAD conference presented by Kwame Nkrumah University of Science and Technology (KNUST) in Kumasi, Ghana in 2017. This was the first time this event was presented as a conference not a symposium. The conference continued using the eight commissions that had guided the 2014 conference. This was also an exciting time when the World Health Organisation (WHO) Global Cooperation on Assistive Technology (GATE) programme was implemented by

WHO with the intention that WHO member countries could improve in their countries access to high quality, affordable assistive technology for people with varying disabilities, diseases and age-related conditions. We as AfriNEAD, wanted to highlight that without affordable, accessible and quality assistive technology (AT) in the region, inclusion will just be a hearsay.

5.6.6 *Disability Unplugged—Beyond Conventions and Charters: What Really Matters to Persons with Disabilities in Africa*

Disability unplugged—*Beyond Conventions and Charters: what really matters to persons with disabilities in Africa* was the theme for the sixth conference that was held in Cape Town, South Africa in 2020. As a result of COVID-19 and lockdowns, the conference was held virtually. As the network continued to learn from previous research and deliberations at previous conferences, and in line with the global realization and prioritization of the area of assistive technology in affording access, dignity and equality to persons with disabilities (core principles of the UNCRPD), a new commission on assistive technology was introduced at this conference. A decision was made to do away with the research evidence commission from the previous conferences as it was felt it was better being covered in the plenary.

5.6.7 *"Positioning AfriNEAD: Rolling Out Disability Research in Africa"*

The theme for the 7th AfriNEAD conference: *Positioning AfriNEAD: Rolling out Disability Research in Africa* was about experiences and ideas on how AfriNEAD could be better positioned to achieve its quest of being a regional research network for realization of rights of persons with disability in Africa. This title required AfriNEAD to reflect on its organic strength and position in Africa and its ability to face the challenges of the day regarding disability research. AfriNEAD aimed for evidence-based solutions to actions in disability work and to map a plan, a blueprint for going forward.

5.7 Presentation of Seven AfriNEAD Conferences from 2007 to 2023

This section presents the process of organizing and hosting each of the seven AfriNEAD conferences as well as conference outcomes, lessons and impact on AfriNEAD.

5.7.1 The Stellenbosch University Symposium on Evidence-to-Action in Disability (SSEAD)

As earlier explained, the first AfriNEAD conference was hosted by Stellenbosch University in Cape Town, South Africa. At that time the AfriNEAD conferences were known as Symposia. During the hosting of this conference, the AfriNEAD Secretariat was the main driver of the conference planning as there was still a need to have people linked to the network who could support AfriNEAD to set up a conference organizing committee.

We also hired a conference hosting company that was based in our faculty to assist the Secretariat. At that time the AfriNEAD Secretariat consisted of Ms Natalie Melling-Williams, Ms Siphokazi Gcaza and Prof Gubela Mji. These three people with the support of Prof Mac MacLachlan, who was at that time a visiting Professor at the Division of Disability and Rehabilitation Studies (DDRS) and was part of the people that played a leading role in the organization of the conference.

We also needed to seek support internally from Stellenbosch University, Stellenbosch, South Africa. The first people we held meetings with were the late Vice Chancellor Prof Russel Botman and Deputy Vice Chancellor for Research at that time, Dr Engelbrecht. Both were supportive of the idea behind AfriNEAD but felt that we needed to go ahead and present the planned conference to ensure that the idea behind AfriNEAD had a following. They provided financial support for the first AfriNEAD conference. We were also supported by Prof Volmink, who at that time was the Assistant Dean for Research at the Medicine and Health Science Faculty. We also connected with Departments that were involved in Disability Research and two of these were the Department of Education (Prof Estelle Swart) and Psychology (Prof Leslie Swartz). By this time, we had also been conducting discussions with Dr Mzolisi Toni from Disabled people South Africa (DPSA) who further linked us with the Chairpersons of the African Decade, Mr AK Dube, and that of Southern

Africa Federation for the Disabled (SAFOD), the late Mr Alexander Phiri. These disability stakeholders all supported and affirmed the idea behind AfriNEAD. It was important to link with Provincial Government Departments and at that time Ms Marie Hendricks chaired the Disability Desk at the Premiers Office in the Western Cape Government, South Africa. We also approached her, and she gave her full support behind AfriNEAD. We further expanded our net by approaching Mr Vincent Daniels from the Society for the Blind, Western Cape, South Africa. Upon further dialogue with the research unit at our Faculty, the Faculty for Medicine and Health Science, we were questioned about the lack of inclusion of business stakeholders. Though we wrote to the business stakeholders we knew, only Old Mutual, Western Cape South Africa, responded and agreed to send a representative to the conference. Old Mutual further offered one day for this representative to work on AfriNEAD-related matters in the following year.

The post conference reflections from the Chairperson of the conference organizing committee shows that SSEAD conference was a successful endeavour. The conference hoped initially to contribute to efforts to bridge the Evidence-Policy-Practice gaps in disability throughout the region in Africa. The conference further intended to initiate dialogue on how to address the challenges around translating disability-related research into evidence-based advocacy, policy development and practice, to realize the rights of persons with disabilities in the pan-African context. The ethos of the conference was to develop a multi-perspective and interdisciplinary approach to addressing problems facing persons with disabilities, in a serious attempt to develop genuine partnerships at the core of the disability research-policy-action interface. Finally, the conference aimed to attract disability activists, disabled people's organizations, non-governmental organizations, policymakers, practitioners, researchers and academics from throughout Africa, including many disabled participants, to come together and dialogue on how to realize the rights of persons with disabilities in the region.

There was a good response from the different stakeholders who later became the grassroots base for AfriNEAD. The approach of choosing key disability drivers in the region was strategic (Dr Toni: Chairperson at that time for Disabled People South Africa (DPSA), Mr Phiri: Chairperson for Southern Africa Federation for the Disabled (SAFOD) and Mr Dube: Chairperson for the African Decade for persons with Disabilities now known as African Disability Alliance (ADA). During contesting debates in the conference, these stakeholders were able to assist in developing a bridge between persons with disabilities and researchers, highlighting that honest conversations are critical to move forward, but that these conversations should not divide us as we all have one goal which was the realization of rights of persons with disabilities in the region. There was good attendance of regional and international stakeholders. It is important to mention that Irish Aid assisted in bringing sixteen (16) persons with disabilities and disability activists from African countries that were affiliated with AfriNEAD. We were fortunate to have the previous President of Ireland, Honourable Marie Robertson, who gave a keynote address highlighting the big task that AfriNEAD has taken on and quoting from the UNCRPD article 31 of the need for high-income countries to assist low-income countries in implementing the Convention (Honourable Marie Robertson, 2007). The last aspect to be addressed by this conference was the development of a governing structure for AfriNEAD. Below under 5.7.2 the second AfriNEAD conference titled the ABC of Research Evidence-to-Action: putting UNCRPD principles in action for rights-based change is discussed as follows:

5.7.2 The ABC of Research Evidence-to-Action: Putting UNCRPD Principles into Action for Rights-Based Change Conference

This conference was hosted in 2009. At this time the conferences were still called symposia. It was the first time that we used commissioners/ research areas that were an outcome of compressing the 50 articles of the UNCRPD.

This again was a conference organized mainly by the AfriNEAD Secretariat. The only difference to the first was that we brought in a disability activist (Dr Washeila Sait) to assist with organizing the conference. The conference was held at the Lagoon Beach Hotel in Milnerton, Cape Town, South Africa. Since this was the second AfriNEAD conference, the Secretariat had learnt from the previous conference in 2007 on how to do fund raising for the conference. By this time, AfriNEAD, through partnerships, had managed to secure a sizeable research project grant on African Policy on Disability and Development (APODD) that was led by Prof Mac MacLachlan from Trinity in Dublin Ireland, and the lead researchers from South Africa were Mr AK Dube from ADA and Prof Gubela Mji from the Division of Disability and Rehabilitation Studies (DDRS). We were also funded by Stellenbosch University, Stellenbosch, South Africa and the Minister for Children, Women and Persons with Disabilities from the South African Government. This was also the first time that AfriNEAD decided that the conference would end with a celebration of the International Day for persons with disabilities and the aim of this was to share the celebration with regional and international stakeholders who would still be in Cape Town, South Africa. The celebration of the International Day for persons with disabilities was held at the Coetzenberg sport centre, at Stellenbosch University, Stellenbosch, South Africa, and the main key speakers were the late Prof Russel Botman previous Vice Chancellor for Stellenbosch University and the Deputy President of South Africa, who at that time was Mr Kgalema Motlanthe.

This conference was opened by Honourable Minister Noluthando Mayende-Sibiya, the Minister of Women, Children and People with Disabilities, Republic of South Africa. The conference was well-attended and managed to pull together AfriNEAD stakeholders thereby fulfilling AfriNEAD aspirations. We were pleased to see the broad spectrum of stakeholders that attended especially those from the African region and the international world. In this conference there was a deeper level of engagement, enthusiasm and participation of the AfriNEAD membership. As earlier mentioned, this was the first time AfriNEAD used fifty compressed articles from the UNCRPD. Though this might have been a bit overwhelming for some people, we believed however, that it was necessary to expose the AfriNEAD delegates and researchers to the complexities of the issue of equity within the disability field and the need for researchers to see disability as a social construct, in order to understand the multi-faceted approach that research evidence will have to take to bridge the gap between evidence and practice.

A few concerns were expressed during debates regarding some identity issues in respect of AfriNEAD: is AfriNEAD an activist meeting or a research meeting? It was concluded that research is not a black box, a bit more of a rainbow box, and researchers are a rainbow nation. All of us have important roles to play in disability research evidence. We must not be scared to have different identities and roles.

Some of the critical questions were related to research evidence about qualitative and quantitative methodologies. The conclusion was that we need to be willing to swing the pendulum to connect with all the different facets of research that could assist, from small qualitative research studies to large-scale studies (such as surveys) that provide information. Another aspect raised was the need to continue reflecting on the link between poverty and disability and the meaning of this in terms of research methodologies and the use of appropriate instruments, especially in indigenous communities.

Although earlier conflicts picked up in the first conference had improved and there was better focus on the agenda at hand on how research evidence can assist in realizing the rights of persons with disabilities, there were still under-currents of pulling at different angles. It was at this time that AfriNEAD chairperson concluded that this level of mistrust would not quickly disappear. She also felt that as the network was being built, it might be worth using some of the African principles and concepts that could assist calming the waves that were blighting the network. Some of these principles are: Uhambo aluqgitywa ngemini enye (you do not finish a journey in one day) and Ubude abuphangwa (you cannot hurry to be tall). These principles and concepts and their implication for AfriNEAD will be discussed in Chapter 9.

There was a sense that Ubuntu and how it is interpreted and practiced by different nations and worlds could be shared amongst these groups of people that are united by the research purpose. Maybe during this process, it can become clear that we do not have the "them" and "us", but "all of us" ideology.

Despite these challenges we were grateful for the Southern Africa Federation for the Disabled (SAFOD) offer to host the AfriNEAD 2011 symposium under the leadership of Mr Alexander Phiri. When we suggested that conference attendees should bid to host the conference, only Mr Phiri offered. When the AfriNEAD Chairperson shared the need to develop an African Journal of Disability—Mr Phiri strongly supported this and suggested that Professor Leslie Swartz become the first Editor in Chief of this journal. Below under 5.7.3 the third AfriNEAD conference with the title: Building Communities of Trust: Evidence-to-Action in Disability Research is discussed as follows:

5.7.3 *Building Communities of Trust: Evidence-to-Action in Disability Research conference*

This third AfriNEAD conference was hosted at Victoria Falls in Zimbabwe in 2011. It was a collaboration between AfriNEAD and SAFOD. This was the first time that the conference was hosted outside South Africa. There was a great excitement in getting ready for this conference as AfriNEAD would be fulfilling one of its objectives for the first time—that is hosting an AfriNEAD conference outside South Africa. Unfortunately, Mr Alexandria Phiri the Chairperson of SAFOD had died by the time the conference was hosted.

AfriNEAD's intention was that once the conference started being hosted outside South Africa, the AfriNEAD Secretariat would visit the hosting country before the conference to give support with conference preparations. The first visit to Bulawayo in Zimbabwe, where SAFOD offices were situated, was in 2010. This visit went smoothly as Mr Phiri was still alive. He also assisted the AfriNEAD Secretariat in shouldering the costs related to accommodation. The second visit was in July 2011, three months after Mr Phiri had died. This visit was linked to the need for the AfriNEAD Secretariat to evaluate whether it would still be feasible to host the conference as planned because many within the Governing Structure of AfriNEAD were suggesting that the conference be postponed to a later date. When the Secretariat visited SAFOD, although grieving for their late leader, they found an organization that was resolute to host the conference.

The conference was well attended by Zimbabweans as well as regional and international delegates. There were a lot of familiar faces from the previous conferences. It appeared that the network was starting to develop a following. There were also eager new faces that were ready to bring new life to the network. We also want to thank the Foundation for Scientific and Industrial Research (SINTEF) in Norway for ensuring that persons with disabilities from Zimbabwe could attend the conference. We are also grateful for the financial support that was given by Stellenbosch University, Stellenbosch, South Africa.

The theme and the programme of this conference offered food for thought and Dr Rachel Kachaje supported and guided the conference with a keynote address on this area. It was humbling to listen to some of our delegates within the conference who did not shy away from sensitive topics such as disability and sexuality, reminding us that persons with disabilities are sexual beings, as the book "Look at me" which was donated to all conference delegates by Dr Marlene Le Roux highlighted this issue. On the other hand, some of the papers shared concerns about disabled women who were undermined, ignored and abused sexually.

The African Journal of Disability was inaugurated during this conference, opening an avenue for papers from this conference and beyond to be published. It was the first time that there were countries that offered to bid for the 2014 conference; these countries were Ghana,

Namibia and Malawi. As it appeared that the network was starting to consolidate its membership, there was a warning from the chairperson that the network must link with other smaller networks doing the same work and not become too cosy. It was heartwarming to see the twenty SAFOD research trainees during breaks gathering information on how delegates were experiencing the conference. Below under 5.7.4 the fourth AfriNEAD conference with the title: intensifying disability research and practice to achieve the MDGs in Africa: our experience and aspirations for the future is discussed as follows:

5.7.4 Intensifying Disability Research and Practice to Achieve the MDGs in Africa: Our Experience and Aspirations for the Future

The University of Malawi was the only country that was able to send a completed bid document to the AfriNEAD conference. This conference was hosted at the Sun and Sands Resort in MangochI in Malawi in 2014. The bid document suggested that the theme of the conference was to be "Intensifying disability research and practice to achieve the MDGs in Africa: our experience and aspirations for the future". The lead person for the conference organizing committee was Professor Allister Munthali from the University of Malawi in Zomba, Malawi.

The intention of the AfriNEAD Secretariat was to visit the conference organizing committee twice. In the first visit, we held a successful whole day meeting with the committee. After this for the whole week we visited Government Departments and DPOs. At that time Dr Rachel Kachaje was the Minister for Elderly and persons with disabilities. We visited many DPOs as Prof Allister Munthali was knowledgeable about all these stakeholders and was a good networker. Lastly, we visited the hosting Resort, Mangochi—even here there was willingness to adjust according to what we saw as aspects related to accessibility. As we were driving to the airport, we were not sure if we were going in the correct direction. We saw a group of three boys, and one had disability—what humbled us was that though the disabled boy was shuffling on his buttocks for walking as he did not have a wheelchair—the abled bodied boys allowed the disabled boy to be the one who ultimately reached the car to give us directions—they waited until he could reach the car to participate. This inclusion and patience of these boys at grassroots level humbled us.

Reflections from the Chairperson of the Conference Organizing Committee attest to a well-attended conference with over 200 conference delegates. One could see in the conference the various AfriNEAD stakeholders. There was the Minister of Gender, Children, Disability and Social Welfare, Patricia Kaliati and the Deputy President for Disability People International Ms Rachel Kachaje, the President of CBM, Dave McComiskey, Prof Usef Chikte the Executive Head of the Department of Interdisciplinary Health Sciences at the Medicine and Health Science Faculty, Stellenbosch University, South Africa. We were also fortunate to have the Deputy Director-General-Strategic Program from the Premier's office of the Western Cape Government in South Africa Dr. Laurie Platzky. Additionally, SAFOD had a new Chairperson Mr Mussa Chiaula, who also attended the conference.

We were proud of the AJOD journal (www.ajod.org) which in this conference showcased the journal's 1st Special issue that emerged from the conference in 2011. The journal was now an accredited journal in South Africa. The call to the researchers and practitioners was to prepare papers for the 2nd AJOD Special issue. AfriNEAD had its website ready www.sun.ac.za/AfriNEAD.

It was with joy that Kwame Nkrumah University of Science and Technology, Kumasi, Ghana, expressed a need to host the 5th AfriNEAD conference without going through the process of bidding with other countries, the Governing Body of AfriNEAD agreed to this on condition that they complete the bidding document to demonstrate their readiness to host the conference. Below under 5.7.5 the fifth AfriNEAD conference with the title: Disability and Inclusion in Africa: The role of assistive technology is discussed as follows:

5.7.5 "Disability and Inclusion in Africa: The Role of Assistive Technology"

This conference was hosted at the Kwame Nkrumah University of Science and Technology KNUST in Kumasi, Ghana in 2017. As earlier mentioned, this conference and its theme was influenced by the WHO initiative on assistive technology (AT) with the goal of making governments that are aligned with WHO aware that there could never be comprehensive inclusion for persons with disabilities without ensuring that each person with disability has appropriate, affordable and accessible ATs. The DDRS at Stellenbosch University, Stellenbosch, South

Africa, together with the Disability Studies Unit at the University of Cape Town, Cape Town, South Africa, has spent some time assisting Kwame Nkrumah University of Science and Technology (KNUST) in Kumasi, Ghana, to develop a Bachelor of Science (BSc) in Disability and Rehabilitation Studies and a Masters in Disability Studies. As AfriNEAD Secretariat, we hoped that the KNUST conference theme would include something related to AT. They came up with the above conference theme. We visited KNUST twice and on the second visit KNUST was ready to host the conference. Below are reflections from the Chairperson of the conference organizing committee Prof Anthony Edusei on the process of organizing to host the conference that happened in KNUST.

The conference was organized at the University campus of KNUST, which offered the opportunity to have reduced rates for facilities used. The hosting of the 5th AfriNEAD conference coincided with the hosting of the 7th College of Health Sciences Scientific Conference, and the two events were combined as the 7th College of Health Scientific Conference and the 5th AfriNEAD Conference with the AfriNEAD theme. KNUST had a strong group for the conference organizing committee and informed us that the conference would be hosted in the new accessible engineering Department. This was a pride for them to showcase this new accessible building that was near their fully accessible Disability Unit.

The opportunity to host the 5th AfriNEAD Conference was offered by KNUST after the 4th AfriNEAD Conference held in 'Sun and Sand' Hotel in Mangochi, Malawi, in 2014. Planning for the 5th AfriNEAD conference started in earnest from the beginning of 2015. Membership of the planning committee comprised a standing Scientific Committee, appointed by the College of Health Sciences to plan its biennial Scientific Conference. Other members included some members of the Department of Community Health of the School of Medical Sciences and the School of Public Health, KNUST and representatives of the Ghana Federation of Disability Organizations, Ghana Blind Union, National Council on Persons with Disability, NGOs in Disability and Ministry of Gender, Children and Social Protection. The committee was co-chaired by Dr. T. B. Kwoffie of the College of Health Sciences, KNUST and Dr. Obeng Asamoa of the Ghana Blind Union. The activities of the local planning committee were fully complemented by the AfriNEAD chairperson and the Secretariat at Stellenbosch University in South Africa.

The entire event comprised an impressive official opening, which was attended by dignitaries, including the representative of Otumfuo

Osei Tutu II, Asantehene and Chancellor of KNUST, Minister of Gender, Children and Social Protection, representing His Excellency Nana Addo Dankwa Akuffo-Addo, the President of the Republic of Ghana, AfriNEAD Chairperson, Prof. Gubela Mji, Pro-Vice Chancellor of KNUST, Ashanti Regional Minister, Mayor of Kumasi City, Honourable Madam Hellen Zille Premier of Western Cape Provincial Government, Republic of South Africa, Prof. Yusuf Chikte, representing the Vice Chancellor of Stellenbosch University, Stellenbosch, South Africa, Prof. T. Agbenyega, Provost of the College of Health Sciences, KNUST and several other dignitaries including some core group members of AfriNEAD.

The planned activities for the conference comprised keynote presentations, plenary and scientific sessions. The keynote addresses presented during the opening featured the perspective of a renowned educationist, a seasoned orthopaedic surgeon, an experienced disability and rehabilitation practitioner with a vast experience in orthotics and prostheses, two key personalities from SAFOD (Dr Rachel Kachaje and Mr Mussa Chiwaula) and one person from the Western Cape Network for persons with disabilities (Mr Rustim Ariefdien) with a wealth of experience on disability issues, as persons with disability themselves. The conference also featured a workshop on Scientific Writing, facilitated by Prof. Leslie Swartz, a project meeting by researchers and workshops by Foundation for Scientific and Industrial Research (SINTEF) Norway. Additionally, a workshop on assistive devices was facilitated by Dr. Diane Bell from the WHO GATE Project.

The conference was a well-attended three-day event, fully packed with stimulating, educative and useful information that will propel the needed paradigm shift when it comes to the inclusion of disability issues in human developmental agenda to facilitate the inclusive society, we so desire. Below under 5.7.6 the sixth AfriNEAD conference with the title: Disability unplugged—beyond conventions and Charters: what really matter to persons with disabilities in Africa is discussed as follows:

5.7.6 Disability Unplugged—Beyond Conventions and Charters: What Really Matters to Persons with Disabilities in Africa

The conference would again be hosted by Stellenbosch University, Stellenbosch, Cape Town in 2020 after being hosted in three countries outside South Africa. These countries were: Zimbabwe 2011, Malawi

2014 and Ghana 2017. For the AfriNEAD Secretariat the return of the conference to Stellenbosch University was a big opportunity to take stock of AfriNEAD and the growth that the network has achieved by hosting the conference in other countries.

The 6th AfriNEAD conference was a celebration of the coming home of AfriNEAD conference, after successfully hosting the conferences in other African countries. The COVID-19 pandemic created a crisis that paralysed the global family. This crisis shone a spotlight on pre-existing social inequalities with certain groups being doubly affected by the pandemic. Persons with disabilities who already had baseline burdens of disease at higher rates than those who are not disabled, including poverty and challenges within our health systems, that are not conducive to their needs, were deeply affected. Hence, as the AfriNEAD conference organizing committee, we decided to continue to host the conference. At this time the AfriNEAD Secretariat was able to gather a conference organizing committee. Initially, the Chairperson for this Committee was Dr Nico Elema, but due to work pressures, this role was handed to Dr Marcia Lyner-Cleophas. It was clear then that this would be a virtual conference, and we were fortunate to be joined by Edit Micro Systems and their Tech Team in Table view, South Africa. It was the first time that they hosted a virtual conference of an international nature. They graciously did this at no cost—we will forever be grateful to this organization for their support.

The original plan was to host the conference at the Artscape—Cape Town's main centre for the performing arts, in a face-to-face mode and at no cost. A huge thank you goes to Dr Marlene Le Roux for this generous offer. The Chairperson of AfriNEAD at that time also extended gratitude to the Stellenbosch University Disability Unit and the Western Cape Network for Persons with Disabilities for their support in preparing for the conference. We also would like to thank the Stellenbosch University Rectorate especially Prof Eugene Cloete, Dr Nico Elema and the Premiers Office for their financial support and believing in the vision of this conference from a research and practice perspective, in the field of disability.

In preparing for the conference, we also knew that this would be a time for internal reflection by Stellenbosch University (SU), Stellenbosch South Africa, on the ground covered in creating an inclusive University. It was within this endeavour that the following actions were taken: (a) tabling of monthly publication prepared by and presented by past students with disability, reflecting on their experience of being a student with disability at SU, (b) the awarding of an Honorary Doctorate Degree in Social Sciences to Ms Rachel Kachaje—unfortunately by the time it was awarded, she already had passed away, (c) the tabling of sign language and disability seminars with reports from these seminars presented to the University management for their action.

Planning for the 2020 conference started in earnest in 2019, prior to the outbreak of the COVID-19 pandemic. Nobody could have predicted how the world would be impacted at that stage. In December 2019, Stellenbosch University (SU) also declared the year 2020 as the Year of Persons with Disabilities where we planned to pause and reflect on our success and as well explore the areas of disability inclusion that needed improvement. During 2020, Rachel Kachaje, a stalwart in the world of disability, sadly passed away. The year 2020 was a tumultuous year indeed!

In conjunction with the Disability Unit (DU), the Transformation Office (TO) and AfriNEAD based at the Division of Disability and Rehabilitation studies (DDRS), we planned a range of reflective activities, such as a Human Rights lecture in March, articles published by staff and students with disabilities in the SU media, Casual Day activities according to the 2020 theme, and seminars, to name a few. These activities culminated in the 6th AfriNEAD conference 1–2 December 2020, followed by the International Day for Persons with Disabilities on 3 December 2020. The articles written by SU previous students were also showcased in the conference booklet.

A conference organizing committee was established early in 2019 which consisted of staff members from the Disability Unit, the Transformation Office, Western Cape Network for Persons with Disabilities, AfriNEAD chairperson and secretariat, staff from the DDRS, selected NGOs in Cape Town and the private sector willing to support the success of AfriNEAD and its conference.

The privilege to host the return of the African Network for Evidence-to-Action in Disability (AfriNEAD) conference to South Africa in December 2020 came amidst a historically unexpected context, the COVID-19 pandemic. The conference was to be held at Artscape, a premier theatre in the City of Cape Town.

The 6th AfriNEAD conference was finally held on a virtual Zoom platform, with the digital back-up support of Edit Micro, a digital, hardware- and software Company in Table view, Cape Town, which specializes in assistive technologies for people with disabilities. We were very grateful for the offer of Artscape for the physical venue, but large groups in one space was not allowed due to the COVID-19 pandemic. This meant that the costs of the conference as initially established was drastically reduced to virtual participation costs only.

Abstracts were received and 53 were accepted. All presenters were encouraged to do pre-recordings of their presentations, given the difficulties that could arise with digital and live presentations. The virtual conference opening had everybody at the edge of their seats, as if they were in the Artscape Theatre (where they were meant to be) waiting for a performance. The big difference was that most of us were sitting in the comfort of our homes or offices across the world. Delegates came from Norway, Congo, Malawi, Zimbabwe, Cape Town, USA and many others—a Total of 31 countries (see conference report for 2020).

The virtual event was opened by Prof Gubela Mji, chairperson of AfriNEAD. The first session for the first day was chaired by Dr Mzolisi Toni. The moderator Ms Luigia Nicholas assisted in linking up the different sections of the conference. The opening of the second day was chaired by Mr Rustim Ariefdien. We appreciate the many persons that assisted in chairing the many sections of the conference. Ms Hillary Lane chaired the 3rd day. The conference was also supported by representatives from WHO Geneva and African Region (Mr Chapal Khasnabis, Dr Mac MacLachlan and Dr Aissatou Sougou) and Ms Irene Esambo, Minister for people with disability from the Democratic Republic of Congo (DRC). Ms Charlotte McClain-Nhlapo, the Global Disability Advisor for the World Bank Group delivered a speech in honour of and celebrating the life of Ms. Rachel Kachaje.

The conference comprised presentations introduced by the many chairpersons, who in turn were introduced by a moderator. Presentations were mostly recorded. Most recordings had captions added and South African Sign Language interpretation was available during the conference. French interpretation was available as needed. Apps such as Otter.ai and Live Transcribe was recommended where participants needed speech-to-text conversion during the conference. Presentations that were not part of plenary were organized according to the AfriNEAD thematic areas. We have managed to have some of the conference presentations available online (www.sun.ac.za/AfriNEAD).

Presentations were done by various key researchers and notable people with disability, civil society and NGO's and various universities across the globe. Details are evident in the conference programme. No research writing workshop took place during this virtual conference given the challenges this could present. The virtual conference had a registration of 174 people and was attended by 156 people, and was considered a successfully executed conference, given the novelty of doing an AfriNEAD event in completely virtual format for the first time.

It is envisaged that a hybrid form of the conference be explored going forward: virtual and face-to-face. This would likely attract the traditional and wider audience and would allow for a wider economic range of participation. Bringing into the fold younger researchers and participants need to be endeavoured as we charter the way forward. The digital age and new ways of thinking about the world is fostered in this way. Below under 5.7.7 the seventh AfriNEAD conference with the title: Positioning AfriNEAD: Rolling out disability research in Africa is discussed as follows:

5.7.7 "Positioning AfriNEAD: Rolling Out Disability Research in Africa"

The 7th AfriNEAD conference in 2023 was again hosted in Cape Town at Artscape. This was the second conference that was held in Cape Town South Africa after three conferences that were held in Zimbabwe, Malawi and Ghana. The intention was that at the end of this conference there would be a bidding process for countries that intend to host the 8th AfriNEAD conference in 2026.

AfriNEAD conference organizing usually starts the year before hosting the conference. At this juncture it was easy for AfriNEAD to organize a conference organizing committee as AfriNEAD had a local following both within Stellenbosch University and the Cape Town community. There were also colleagues from the region and internationally who joined the conference organizing committee. The Stellenbosch University Disability Unit, the Western Cape Network for Persons with disabilities and Edit Micro Systems played a pivotal role in sending people to participate in organizing this conference. For Chairperson for the conference organizing committee, AfriNEAD Chairperson asked Dr Lyner–Cleophas who chaired the previous conference. This was a hybrid conference and was held at the Artscape theatre for onsite participants. We are thankful to Dr Marlena Le Roux for assisting AfriNEAD to host the conference at Artscape at no cost. Again, Edit Micro Systems assisted with the virtual component of the conference to host a successful conference. We also would like to extend gratitude to the Rectorate of Stellenbosch University for again endorsing and supporting this conference and AfriNEAD. Our greatest gratitude goes to the following organizations for their support: Wes Gro, Irish Embassy, World Bank, Premier of the Western Cape and Edit Micro System.

The return home of AfriNEAD conferences in 2020 gave AfriNEAD space to strengthen some of the critical areas such as the business plan and the development of the Governing document for AfriNEAD. We also went through a time for internal reflection by Stellenbosch University (SU) on the ground covered in creating an inclusive University. Other related activities to the hosting of the conference by Stellenbosch University was the awarding of Honorary Doctorate degree to Dr Charlotte McClean-Nhlapho.

The conference chairperson's report highlighted the following about the conference: The African Network for Evidence-to-Action in Disability (AfriNEAD) conference held its 7th conference in Cape Town, South Africa. The 6th conference was also held in Cape Town, but due to the 2020 global Coronavirus pandemic that broke out, it was held virtually. The decision to hold the 7th conference as hybrid (both virtual and in person) in Cape Town was made to accommodate people who could not physically come to Cape Town for the conference. This was indeed the case, and the conference took place from 29 to 30 November and 1 and 3 December 2023 (3 December became a sight-seeing day for delegates).

Approximately 220 delegates registered for the conference or joined online. The countries that were represented are: Belgium, Botswana, Cameroon, Canada, Democratic Republic of Congo, Ethiopia, Ghana, India, Ireland, Kazakhstan, Kenya, Malawi, Mauritius, Mozambique, Namibia, Niger, Nigeria, Norway, Rwanda, Somalia, South Africa, Tanzania, The Gambia, Uganda, United Kingdom, United States, Zambia and Zimbabwe. Conference IT was done by Edit Micro in Cape Town and generally went very well. A highly competent team ran this conference for a second time (2020 was their first).

The next AfriNEAD conference will be contested through an application process which was shared with the core AfriNEAD group. We look forward to that conference at a location other than South Africa, but still on the African continent.

Young and emerging researchers are entering the fold and promise to bring along fresh inspiration to AfriNEAD. The change in the chairperson of AfriNEAD goes together with the change in leadership of the Division for Disability and Rehabilitation Studies. The newly elected incumbent,

Prof Lieketseng Ned, replaced the outgoing Prof Gubela Mji of both the DDRS and AfriNEAD and we look forward to supporting and strengthening AfriNEAD in its future endeavours as it grows from strength to strength.

A recommendation is that conference planning be outsourced to a reputable conference organizing committee that will work in close collaboration with the AfriNEAD Secretariat, and that is au fait with disability-related conference with its many nuances. Matters such as billing, invoicing, bookings, conference reception area, email and other communications with delegates to name a few should be done by professional people that are au fait with planning disability-related conference. Meticulous administration is vital for a smooth-running conference to the end. Attention must also be paid to the catering, as this is an important element of any conference.

The leadership of AfriNEAD and all committee leads are hugely thanked for their commitment and expertise since the 2007 conference. They are wished only the best as they charter the waters ahead. Below under 5.5 is a summary of conference outcomes and lessons learnt from the seven AfriNEAD conferences hosted from 2007 to 2023.

5.8 Summary of Conference Outcomes and Lessons Learnt from the Seven AfriNEAD Conferences Hosted from 2007 to 2023

Table 5.8 presents the conference outcomes, lessons learnt and impact on AfriNEAD progress that emerged from the presentation of AfriNEAD conferences starting from the first conference in 2007 and to the last one before the writing of this book in 2023. A more detailed account of this area is presented under 5.7 on presentation of seven AfriNEAD conferences from 2007 to 2023 (Table 5.2).

Some Reflections on Conference Outcomes and Lessons Learnt from the Seven AfriNEAD Conferences Hosted from 2007 to 2023.

Table 5.8 provides an overview of conference outcomes and lessons learnt from the seven AfriNEAD conferences. Since the first AfriNEAD conference in 2007, there has been an upward thread in the development of AfriNEAD. When the Chairperson of AfriNEAD consulted with the Rectorate of Stellenbosch University, at Stellenbosch in South Africa to ask permission and support to initiate the research program on disability

Table 5.2 Summary of conference outcomes and lessons learnt from the seven AfriNEAD conferences hosted from 2007 to 2023

Conference theme	*Conference outcomes*	*Lessons learnt*	*Impact on AfriNEAD progress*
The first AfriNEAD conference in Cape Town South Africa November 2007: The Stellenbosch University Symposium on Evidence- to-Action in Disability (SSEAD)	- The successful presentation of the SSEAD conference and development of a network - Development of the Governing structure of the Network - Publication of conference outcomes in the International Journal of Disability and Rehabilitation - Funds left over from hosting conference for running AfriNEAD Secretariat.	- Importance of choosing Gate keepers that are relevant for the sustainability of the network - When aiming to develop honest, trustful and lasting relationships, it is important to allow difficult challenging conversations to happen	In this first conference, both the conference outcomes and lessons learnt gave AfriNEAD a stepping stone for building the network as AfriNEAD could leverage on the three conference outcomes, i.e.: The developed network, the governing structure and availability of funds to drive the network
The second AfriNEAD conference in Cape Town South in November 2009: The ABC of Research Evidence-to-Action: putting UNCRPD principles into action for rights-based change conference	- Increased conference participants - Launch of Disability research manual: "Doing disability research: A practical guide to disability research in Africa" - Mr Phiri to host the conference in Zimbabwe - Plans to develop disability journal with an already identified editor in chief - AfriNEAD celebrated the 3rd of December together with persons with disabilities	- Continued dialogue was still necessary with AfriNEAD stakeholders as there was still an unease in working together - Identity issues and issues related to research evidence kept emerging during discussions, including whether research methodologies that have been developed in the Global North are suitable for the African region	- In this second conference, though the network was growing with regard to the membership and aspects related to research evidence and the opportunity to host the conference outside South Africa, there was a clarion call to address issues of relationships between researchers and persons with disabilities, hence the decision by the AfriNEAD Secretariat for the third AfriNEAD conference to focus on building trust amongst the network membership

(continued)

Table 5.2 (continued)

Conference theme	*Conference outcomes*	*Lessons learnt*	*Impact on AfriNEAD progress*
The third AfriNEAD conference in Zimbabwe in November 2011: Building Communities of Trust: Evidence -to - Action in Disability Research	- The successful hosting of AfriNEAD conference outside South Africa - The new faces that were joining the AfriNEAD network - African Journal of Disability (AJOD) ready to accept manuscripts - Donated book on disabled women and their sexuality by Dr Le Roux on "Look at me" - African Policy on Disability and Development (APODD) and SANPAD projects contributing to research evidence - SAFOD research trainees' engagement with conference attendees	- There is a need for patience in building the network as at this conference, one could see that AfriNEAD membership was uniting and becoming a family, there was less fighting and more unity - There is a need to continue working on issues of trust	Coming out of the third AfriNEAD conference there was a level of confidence from the network that it can deliver its mandate of building the network membership and production of research evidence The network Governance was also open to dialogue and willing to build trust amongst its membership. The hosting of the conference outside South Africa gave the network confidence that it was starting to be an African network

Conference theme	*Conference outcomes*	*Lessons learnt*	*Impact on AfriNEAD progress*
The fourth AfriNEAD conference in Malawi in November 2014: Intensifying disability research and practice to achieve the MDGs in Africa: our experience and aspirations for the future	- The special issue from the 3rd AfriNEAD conference of 2011 published in the AfriNEAD journal the African Journal of Disability (AJOD) - Emergence and completion of multi-country studies from African Policy on Disability and Development and Equitable projects - The announcement of the AfriNEAD website www.sun.ac.za/AfriNEAD - The attendance of AfriNEAD conference by Ms Laurine Platkzy, the strategist for the Government of the Western Cape	- The important role and product of networking could be seen at play in this country as the key organizing person had managed to draw many Disabled People Organizations from grassroots to attend the conference - It is important to initiate aspects such as the African Journal of Disability that will advance the disability debate as it has started fulfilling one of the AfriNEAD objectives, i.e. to compile and publish a special issue from AfriNEAD conferences - The learning lesson from young boys from Malawi that disability does not mean inability	- The experience that AfriNEAD gained from the fourth conference was how the main conference organizer was able to role play inclusiveness and networking utilizing key disability role players that were based in Malawi - The inauguration of the AJOD in this conference gave opportunity for researchers to have an African disability journal to publish their work - Linking AfriNEAD with Government stakeholders opened opportunity to extend networking for AfriNEAD

(continued)

Table 5.2 (continued)

Conference theme	*Conference outcomes*	*Lessons learnt*	*Impact on AfriNEAD progress*
The fifth AfriNEAD conference in Ghana in November 2017: "Disability and Inclusion in Africa: The Role of Assistive Technology"	- KNUST combined two conferences into one as the 7th College of Health Scientific Conference and the 5th AfriNEAD Conference with the AfriNEAD theme - Development of an advocacy group called 'Advocates for Disability-Friendly KNUST'—AforD-KNUST, in the university - The opportunity for young graduates from the Disability and Rehabilitation Studies Programme of CEDRES to experience an international conference but also to participate as presenters of scientific papers from their original research work	- Everyone gains from improving accessibility as the improvement of accessibility in the building of the engineering department benefited everybody as the conference was held there without hiring a venue outside the University - The hosting of the AfriNEAD conference gave institutions a time to reflect on issues of inclusion and accessibility	- The fifth AfriNEAD conference demonstrated that disability is everybody's business and where possible it is important to try and include as many people as possible to participate in the conference - Hosting AfriNEAD conference in an academic institution assisted to highlight issues of accessibility in that institution and possibility of that institution improve on these areas

Conference theme	*Conference outcomes*	*Lessons learnt*	*Impact on AfriNEAD progress*
The sixth AfriNEAD conference in Cape Town, South Africa in November 2020: Disability unplugged- Beyond Conventions and Charters: what really matters to persons with disabilities in Africa	- To present a successful conference in a virtual format for the first time ever - An African-based slant to evidence and practice-based opportunities was starting to emerge from presentations - Stellenbosch University still demonstrated commitment to AfriNEAD by funding colleagues that were participating in Disability research country working groups from various countries - As build up to the conference, the disability Unit and DDRS presented workshops related to disability - We were also able to award posthumously a Doctorate degree in Social Sciences to Rachel Kachaje	- Conference attendees did not have to be physically present to attend a conference, but the value of face-to-face networking was not undermined - To consider a hybrid format that will attract virtual as well as face-to-face networking and contact, for the next conference	- The hybrid conference offered AfriNEAD future opportunities of hosting conferences virtual -Using virtual means AfriNEAD was able to strengthen the area of Disability research working groups -The awarding of a doctoral degree posthumously to Dr Rachel Kachaje opened opportunities for other people to select persons with disabilities in their own institutions for awarding of honorary degrees

(continued)

Table 5.2 (continued)

Conference theme	*Conference outcomes*	*Lessons learnt*	*Impact on AfriNEAD progress*
The seventh AfriNEAD conference in Cape Town in November 2023: "Positioning AfriNEAD: Rolling out Disability Research in Africa"	- The successful hosting of the hybrid conference - The three countries (Tanzania, Ethiopia and Kenya) that bid to host the AfriNEAD conference in 2026 - The hosting of the workshop on disability researchers in the region - Participation of young people in the conference, giving a sense of continuity	- The need to outsource the conference to a professional conference organizing committee who will work in close collaboration with the Conference Organizing Committee (CoC) to ensure that disability-related conference nuances are addressed	- Participation of younger people in AfriNEAD gave hope for continuity of the network. - There is a need to strengthen the AfriNEAD secretariat for AfriNEAD to comprehensively deliver its mandate

research, the Deputy Vice Chancellor at that time asked the AfriNEAD Chairperson to host a conference to see if there will be any following for this area. The 2007 Stellenbosch Symposium on Evidence-to-Action (SSEAD) was a resounding success, and it was clear by the end of the conference that it is important to build an entity such as AfriNEAD. This was further affirmed by the formulation of the AfriNEAD Governing structure that presented the model that AfriNEAD was suggesting for its constituency (Disability activist, disability researchers, government, business and civil society formations) (Mji et al., 2009; Kachaje et al., 2014).

Given the history of exclusion and oppression of persons with disabilities in Africa, the issue of developing trustful relationships between disability researchers and persons with disabilities took its own time to consolidate (Mji et al., 2011). The role that was played by the Southern Africa Organisation for the Disabled (SAFOD) Research Program whereby the leader of this research program was a person with disabilities also affirmed that persons with disabilities can play different roles in disability research. The issue of developing meaningful relationships was critical in the development of a stable network, hence AfriNEAD Secretariat afforded the third conference the theme: Building communities of Trust with Dr Rachel Kachaje giving a keynote address in this conference to address this issue.

The critical agenda for AfriNEAD was on how research evidence is produced and utilized. Since its inauguration in 2007 there has been an upward thread in disability research in Africa. This has culminated with the production of the African Journal of Disability (AJOD). AJOD-assisted AfriNEAD to develop a platform whereby conference outcomes such as articles now have a platform for publication. As AfriNEAD continued to engage with disability research, disability research scholars such as Botha and Ohajunwa (2024) emphasize the need of seeing a person behind research. Kitchin (2005) asserts that disability research should be wrestled free from academic researchers who are still using traditional research methodologies and, as such, call for the adoption of research strategies that are both emancipatory (seeking 'positive' societal change) and empowering (seeking 'positive' individual change through participation). The participation of SAFOD Research Program scholars in research activities in the 3rd AfriNEAD conference gave hope that though change is slow, persons with disabilities are starting to be central in the production of disability research and now they can play a variety of roles in the production of disability research. This was further affirmed in the 7th AfriNEAD conference whereby young persons with disabilities played a variety of roles in the conference, giving a sense of continuity and stability. This is further affirmed by Botha and Ohajunwa (2024) who maintains that African disability studies scholars are well-placed to disrupt ableism in academic, medical and social spheres, as well as hierarchies within academia, which limit development, mutual growth and respect that in the past has limited participation of persons with disabilities in disability research. Ned et al. (2022) are calling for sustained emancipatory approaches that will help to avoid the reproduction and reinforcement of exclusionary practices that confront persons with disabilities in Africa.

In the 2020 conference it was encouraging to see emerging from presentations African-based slant to evidence and practice-based opportunities. Sefotho (2021) complains of the lack of an African voice in theorizing about disability in the region as what is existing has been developed in the Global North. The development of the network and African Journal of disability creates opportunities for African disability researchers to start documenting experiences in case studies about the lives of persons with disability in Africa. It is hoped that from these case studies, theories related to an African understanding of disability can emerge.

AfriNEAD conferences became a vehicle for funding some of the day-to-day running costs for the AfriNEAD Secretariat. This was not a sustainable funding model. This left AfriNEAD Secretariat constrained to fulfil comprehensively its mandate and quest of being an African network for Evidence to Action in Disability. Below under 5.8 the summary of conference resolutions from the eight thematic areas of the past six AfriNEAD conferences are discussed as follows.

5.9 Summary of Conference Resolutions from the Eight Thematic Areas of the Past Six AfriNEAD Conferences

As earlier stated in Chapter 3, when the AfriNEAD conference is announced, researchers are invited to present abstracts that fit with the thematic areas. The end-product of presentations in each thematic area is a set of resolutions that can be used to highlight the specific disability-related issues to key stakeholders in each field. The conference research outcomes are further consolidated into a special issue published by the African Journal of Disability (Kachaje et al., 2014).

A brief summary of analysis of the resolutions from six AfriNEAD conferences since 2009 was conducted, taking a critical look at the trends and patterns of issues raised across the different commissions (a detailed account is available in AfriNEAD conference reports in the AfriNEAD website www.sun.ac.za/AfriNEAD). The 1st AfriNEAD conference in 2007 was left out of this analysis as the approach of using themes from the UNCRPD only started at the 2009 conference. These resolutions also reveal gaps in research on certain pertinent issues and raise concerns about areas that are recurrent and being highlighted as needing attention at each conference. However, these areas were without enough evidence of change happening to improve the lives of persons with disabilities. The main themes generated from an analysis of the six conference reports are presented below.

5.9.1 Children and Youth with Disabilities

Access to education was raised as the main concern in the theme of Children and Youth with Disabilities. Early intervention and attention to the early childhood development sector that is usually neglected needs more attention. Accessible transport was identified as an important area to be addressed for children and youth to access school and work. The need for teachers who understand disability and inclusive education principles and health professionals who understand disability was raised, especially in rural areas. Availability of assistive devices and technology to facilitate inclusion of children and youth in school, work and other life spaces was also emphasized. Using social cohesion to improve access to services and quality of care for children with disabilities can be achieved through conducting disability community dialogue to create awareness. Ubuntu-informed intervention strategies could assist in collaborating with teachers, and for promoting peer-to-peer support. Research from this commission also shows the importance of training parents and caregivers as non-specialists and part of systems of care.

5.9.2 Education: Early Childhood to Tertiary

Based on the research evidence, it is felt that academic institutions should facilitate the inclusion of disabled students, scholars, researchers and activists in their training and learning programmes as well as incorporate disability issues in all curricula for students and staff inductions. Also, governments should have disability focal points in strategic positions in all government ministries and departments to make education, work and training programmes and policies effective. In-service training of human resource managers, educators and other professions should be prioritized to ensure disability mainstreaming and information and communication technologies (ICT) strategies that take into consideration access for people with disabilities should be prioritized. There is a need to implement peer-to-peer training and parents of children with disabilities (rural areas to be prioritized) must be involved to encourage and develop disability role models. Age requirements for school admission and school-leaving should be flexible to accommodate different needs of learners and vocational training should be linked to work opportunities. For inclusion to happen in schools, training on inclusive education should be compulsory for all teacher trainees, as well as in-service training for those already in the field.

5.9.3 Economic Empowerment

Research on economic empowerment is scarce as shown by the low numbers of papers presented at the AfriNEAD conferences. Recommendations have been made for work to be prioritized in research. Barriers to accessing the work environment which include attitudes, assistive technology, social life and physical space were identified as needing attention. People with disabilities must be given a voice in economic issues and career guidance needs to move to career construction so that more opportunities for employment are available for persons with disabilities. There is also a need to conduct research on why employers are not employing persons with disabilities and deliberate systemic measures need to be established, for example, policies and guidelines for empowering persons with disabilities.

5.9.4 Development Process in Africa: Poverty, Politics and Indigenous Knowledge Systems

This area requires focus on both rural and urban areas as there are also a lot of challenges in urban areas with regard to water, sanitation and hygiene. Women with disabilities experience double discrimination; therefore, there is need for research on their real-life experiences. Implementation of policies and laws can be improved by packaging human rights instruments like laws and policies in various forms accessible to persons with different types of disabilities, e.g. having Acts in Braille and easy to read formats. Access to the judicial system amongst persons with disabilities is critical. The WHO and National guidelines should be standardized and contextualized to be appropriate and relevant to local contexts so that supply matches demand. There is need for understanding of indigenous conceptualizations of assistive technology in African settings to enhance participation of persons with disabilities, and in the process create social theories which enhance understanding of assistive technology in these settings. Additionally, an indigenous knowledge lens should be used when designing policies for the region. This could assist in addressing stigma, for example there is still stigma on those struggling from epilepsy in the region which inhibits disclosure and affects availability of data on epilepsy.

5.9.5 *Health and HIV & AIDS*

Research from this commission shows that the general health and rehabilitation needs of persons and children with disabilities are often ignored and not prioritized. Women with disabilities are often an ideal target for gender-based violence as they are seen as a more vulnerable group. There is also a huge ongoing concern of women being abandoned by their partners after they give birth to a disabled child. Persons with disabilities are not accessing information and treatment on sexual and reproductive health for various reasons and misconceptions still exist about their vulnerability, sexuality and reproductive healthcare needs. Healthcare research does not consider different income brackets and social economic standing. It is also a concern that persons with intellectual disability may suffer from preventable diseases and impairments such as ear infections, dental infections and others.

5.9.6 *Community-Based Rehabilitation*

Recommendations have been made from this commission regarding the role of the government and other stakeholders in supporting and strengthening community-based rehabilitation (CBR) programmes. Governments and Civil Society Organisations (CSOs) should include a mental health perspective within an inclusive holistic approach to disability and develop national CBR and HIV/AIDS implementation strategies, clearly packaged with a resourcing strategy and clear outcome indicators. Governments should formulate disability dedicated budgets with disabled people's organizations (DPOs) monitoring the expenditure and federations/umbrella DPOs should compete less and cooperate more. There is a need for a shift beyond poverty reduction and towards human development. Mental health needs to be considered as part of rehabilitation. There is a need for community-based nutrition education interventions targeting undernourished children.

5.9.7 *Holistic Wellness: Sport, Recreation, Sexuality and Spirituality*

Inclusion of disability sensitization in the curriculum for the training of religious leaders is critical as this has the potential to remove attitudinal barriers, not only in churches but in the larger society. Advocacy campaigns are needed for public education to demystify perceptions regarding marriage for persons with disabilities. High quality contact between persons with and without disabilities is valuable in tackling negative attitudes towards sexuality of persons with disabilities and there is need to remove physical barriers to facilitate such contact. Sport for children with disabilities is essential to give a sense of camaraderie and success and mixing non-disabled and disabled children to play together encourages integration. Communication in one's first language is important in advancing growth of children with disabilities and it needs to be promoted. For young adults, authentic social networks are important in enhancing participation of tertiary students with disabilities. At community level, there is also a need to develop and support persons with disabilities in accessing opportunities to build social networks.

5.9.8 *The Critical Role of Assistive Technology in Facilitating Access to All the Other Rights of Persons with Disabilities in Africa*

Many areas of concern and the need for action have been raised around assistive technology, since the first conference. Assistive technology and its different facets are a recurrent theme in different research commissions. The role of assistive technology in disability inclusive development in Africa needs to be prioritized and governments are expected to enable access to assistive technology to their constituencies. Assistive technology needs to be prioritized in primary healthcare services in the same way preventable practices like vaccinations and medicines are prioritized. There is a need for cultural sensitivity and recognition of indigenous knowledge systems in assistive technology research in Africa. A coordinating body for assistive technology is needed on the continent.

5.10 Aspects Related to Handling of the Resolutions

The area below presents aspects and approaches that could assist the handling of resolutions to move from rhetoric to action.

5.10.1 Packaging and Implementation of Resolutions

Resolutions were made for AfriNEAD to shift from rhetoric to action by working on packaging the recommendations and resolutions for implementation. One statement from the resolutions that captures this recurrent pledge amongst the conference delegates is "*Need to move beyond where we are now, to become ACTION-orientated instead of ongoing debate at a theoretical level*". The arguments and debates occurring at the conferences need to be moved forward to ACTION. The recommendations related to this theme also touched on the issue of *"how to cover the void in-between the conferences"*. The delegates felt that more work must be done in implementation of research evidence and engaging relevant stakeholders so that people do not only wait to attend a conference and forget about the resolutions and recommendations until the next conference.

A question has been asked, *"What have we done with the resolutions except for the publication?"* One response to this question was that research evidence must be well-packaged, for example, writing policy briefs as opposed to research reports; and disseminated to key stakeholders to influence policy and practice.

5.10.2 The Role of the Government

Many of the recommendations tend to be directed towards the governments of African countries as responsible implementers. For example, there is constant recommendation for governments to implement the articles of the UNCRPD in their planning and to address stigmatizing and discriminatory attitudes. For ease of access to resources, it is recommended that governments must create databases for resources available for persons with disabilities in their country. Governments are also called to ensure integration of disability in rural development programmes. Governments should promote home/school partnerships at all levels of education and acknowledge the important role of parents and guardians, by encouraging the establishment of parent support groups, and facilitating support from DPOs and professionals on issues of advocacy, their rights and those of their children, with a special focus on rural areas. Economic empowerment of persons with disabilities must be prioritized by governments employing disabled graduates and giving meaningful salaries not tokenistic salaries. Governments should develop national CBR and HIV/AIDS implementation strategies, clearly packaged with a resourcing strategy and clear outcome indicators. Another recommendation is for governments both in the North and in Africa to support the development of centres of excellence that will facilitate the creativity of persons with disabilities, and manage, disseminate and use research evidence.

5.10.3 *Collaboration and Partnerships Amongst Different Stakeholders*

Partnerships were constantly recognized as prime importance in promoting disability research and its implementation, especially partnerships between researchers, DPO's, governments and the business sector and civil society. The conference delegates agreed in some of the resolutions that all levels of society must be included; from the family, home, village, local community, district and province, using an African community orientation to services and programmes. At the initial conference (symposium), partnerships and collaborations at country level were also recommended and a call made for the African Union to establish a permanent disability commission and to sign agreements that facilitate international cooperation on disability. It was agreed that greater intersectoral collaboration in government must be monitored by DPOs. Also, DPOs must be equal partners in research and service provision. Within the education sector, higher education top management needs more engagement and collaboration with community and disability NGOs.

5.10.4 *Disability Awareness*

Disability awareness has been constantly recognized at all the conferences and in different commissions as a needed strategy to promote inclusion of persons with disabilities. There is a need to educate traditional leaders and interrogate harmful conceptualizations of disability and traditional practices. Persons with disabilities need to be given a voice in matters affecting them by motivating them to speak up and educating them about their rights. More research must be conducted to explore the challenges, beliefs, myths and misconceptions around epilepsy. It is important to break the silence about the sexuality and sexual needs of persons with disabilities and the silence that exists about abuse and discrimination against persons with disabilities. Issues of menstrual hygiene need to be prioritized by governments and other relevant sectors. Intersection of disability stigma, gender and sexuality needs attention.

5.10.5 *Monitoring and Evaluation*

Monitoring and evaluation came up a few times in the conference recommendations and resolutions. For recommended changes to be affected, it was emphasized that policy development must be focused and measures for monitoring of implementation must be put in place. Governments should formulate disability dedicated budgets with disabled people's organizations (DPOs) monitoring the expenditure. Also, monitoring and evaluation must be a continuous action in systems for community-based rehabilitation.

5.11 Overall Successes Aligned with the AfriNEAD Conferences

The AfriNEAD conference has been one of the successful objectives of the network. The conference became a platform whereby key objectives of AfriNEAD were identified and consolidated. The need for the development of a disability journal was identified at the 2009 conference. AfriNEAD then partnered with Kwame Nkrumah University of Science and Technology (KNUST), Kumasi, Ghana and Stellenbosch University, Stellenbosch, South Africa, to establish the African Journal of Disability (AJOD) in 2011, that has successfully published an issue every year since 2012, and it keeps growing from strength to strength.

Following each conference, a special issue dedicated to the conference is published and the special issue editorials present an overview of the conference proceedings and the outcome and resolutions in terms of research evidence.

One of the areas that pose a challenge is the development of Disability Research Country Working Groups (DRCWGs). This area was seen by the AfriNEAD Governing structure as a priority as it will advance the development of AfriNEAD concepts within the African countries affiliated to AfriNEAD. The 2020 COVID-19 and the virtual hosting of the AfriNEAD conference opened opportunities for virtual networking. The AfriNEAD Secretariat used virtual connection to strengthen the development of DRCWGs. There are now nine countries (Ethiopia, Zambia, Zimbabwe, Kenya, Tanzania, Uganda, Ghana, Democratic Republic of Congo and South Africa) committed with representatives from each of them. The Country Working Groups are the hope of the network as they will be able to package the evidence and recommendations from the conferences as relevant to their local contexts (a detailed presentation of DRCWGs is in Chapter 8).

The area of assistive technology (AT) was a recurring theme across the commissions in previous conferences up to 2014, hence it was fitting for the 2017 conference to adopt a theme of assistive technology. A recommendation was made in the 2017 Conference to prioritize research on the role of assistive technology in disability inclusive development in Africa. This was supported by opening a new commission on assistive technology at the 2020 conference through a workshop focusing on collaboration, cohesion and coherence in assistive technology service delivery in Africa. Collaboration, sharing of information and strategies to ensure that assistive technology stakeholders across the continent and wider take ownership of the space, were highlighted as critical and needing to be prioritized. The developments in this area are evident in the exponential increase in research on assistive technology in AfriNEAD-affiliated countries in the past few years (Kahonde & Mji, 2024).

Since its inauguration in 2007, AfriNEAD intended to host two conferences in South Africa consecutively and subsequently, three further conferences to be held consecutively in other African countries. After three conferences hosted in other African countries outside South Africa, two AfriNEAD conferences will again be hosted in South Africa. AfriNEAD has successfully run seven AfriNEAD conferences (four in Cape Town, South Africa: 2007, 2009, 2020, 2023; and the other three in Zimbabwe, 2011, Malawi, 2014 and Ghana, 2017). These conferences managed to draw regional and international participants, and they offer participants opportunities to network.

AfriNEAD utilizes the quarterly newsletter (sent to more than 400 people) and website (www.sun.ac.za/afrinead) to connect with AfriNEAD stakeholders. The Newsletter and the website had played a critical role in planning for an AfriNEAD conference as they are used to announce the conference and to send out a call for abstracts.

5.12 Gaps and Challenges

AfriNEAD is a one-stop place for knowledge sharing about the status of persons with disabilities in Africa. Some of the issues raised in the research papers from all corners of the continent, and presented at the conferences, reveal issues that are seldom talked about or considered as important for persons with disabilities. However, new research touching on different aspects of each theme emerges at each conference before the previous resolutions are acted upon. There is richness in the knowledge shared which requires evidence-to-action.

A gap identified in the recommendations and resolutions is that they are put down and end at *what* needs to be done without going further to define the *how* and *by whom*. There is therefore a need for local activists who use conference resolutions for lobbying and DRCWGs can be a strong partner in this. Hence, AfriNEAD's initiative of establishing DRCWGs to implement the network's model at local country levels is seen as giving hope in this regard. It is also important that the DRCWGs have members who are committed and ready to challenge their governments using evidence from research presented at the conference and other evidence identified in their contexts. These DRCWGs must walk the talk by ensuring that voices of persons with disabilities are heard through including members with different types of disabilities in these groups.

5.13 Reflections from AfriNEAD Coordinator—Walking with AfriNEAD

Ms Hillary Lane has been the AfriNEAD coordinator for more than seven years. One of the core functions of her work was to support the organization of AfriNEAD conferences. She supported the organization of four AfriNEAD conferences (2014: Malawi, 2017: Ghana, 2020, 2023: Cape

Town, South Africa). Below in Table 5.2 is a personal reflection from Ms Hillary Lane AfriNEAD coordinator (Table 5.3).

5.14 Chapter Conclusion

One of AfriNEAD' s objectives and an important tool for networking was the hosting of triennial Africa-wide conferences focusing on issues of interest to assess progress on evidence-to-action and showcase action-to-evidence and to consolidate and take the debate forward on how rights of persons with disabilities could be realized within the region. Through dialogue and debate during conferences, an osmosis of ideas occurred, including the germination and sprouting of completely new ideas. In this manner—though initially there were a lot of contradictions between persons with disabilities and researchers, eventually, the emphasis changed to focus on the agenda at hand which was how to address issues of poverty, access to services and marginalization of persons with disabilities within the region.

AfriNEAD aimed to be an inclusive platform and the adoption of the UNCRPD as a guiding tool for researchers assisted those that were in the past marginalized, to see that debates and outcomes of AfriNEAD conferences are geared towards research evidence that produced data that was aligned with the UNCRPD, which is the document that was produced with and for persons with disabilities. Participation in the network by different stakeholders from local, regional and international contexts assisted its growth. The willingness to debate and enter difficult conversations during symposia/conferences assisted in forging meaningful and sustainable relationships.

The three conferences that were tabled in other African countries (Zimbabwe, 2011; Malawi, 2014; Ghana, 2017) afforded the network further growth and resilience. This gave the network a glimpse of its quest to be an African Network. Coming back to host the conferences at Stellenbosch University (SU), Stellenbosch, South Africa—it was clear that the gaze of the network was focused on the growth of SU as an inclusive university that is conscious of those living at the margins such as students with disabilities, hence the year 2020 was adopted by the institution as a year for persons with disability and during 2020 and 2023 two honorarium doctorate degrees were awarded to persons with disabilities.

Table 5.3 Personal reflection from Ms Hillary Lane AfriNEAD coordinator

Personal reflection from Ms Hillary Lane AfriNEAD coordinator
Each of the four conferences, in which I was privileged to be involved, have been so different! Well, they would have to be, as they were in three different countries
The second AfriNEAD conference was held in Cape Town, and for some reason I gave an address. What struck me there, was how many people attended and that they came from all over the world, and that there was such a strong local support. Whatever AfriNEAD was setting out to do, there was obviously a great need for it
June 2013 was a start of a very exciting journey for me! Before my arrival, AfriNEAD had not previously had a dedicated coordinator and so being available, I was fortunately able to take up the position. I had always wanted to attend university, after leaving school, but for practical reasons this had not been open to me. So, this was a dream come true—being at a university and now in particular, Stellenbosch University
So, my first conference, and the third AfriNEAD conference was held at the Sand 'n Sun hotel in Mangochi, on the shores of Lake Malawi. Our recon visit showed us that there was a good committee driving the event and a good working relationship was established with them
The actual conference in August, attracted people from all over the world. As an organizer there is not much time to participate in the conference as one must be behind the scenes sorting out unplanned eventualities, preparing for the next session, and making sure that the needs and requirements of delegates are met. This also means being on good terms with the hotel manager! In Malawi, a hand basin had to be knocked out of bathroom to provide access for a person in a wheelchair into the shower, or to make sure that delegates who could not push themselves in their wheelchairs, were not forgotten, or that a visually impaired person knew how to get from their room to the dining room. Printing had to be done, which at that time it was not as straightforward as it is now. Also, making sure that people with different dietary needs got what they ordered
The next conference was held in Ghana. As in Malawi, there was a very good team leading the planning for the conference. They also bent over backwards to accommodate us in whatever way they could. On our second visit we were able to fly to Kumasi from Accra in a small aircraft but for the conference we had to hire a vehicle specifically to accommodate people with power wheelchairs. These delegates were later not able to join in the gala dinner as it was totally inaccessible. In both cases, Malawi and Ghana the support for AfriNEAD was unprecedented, which allowed amongst other things the growth and support of AfriNEAD.
Following on from Ghana, the next conference was due to be held in Cape Town, and then Covid 19 struck! The decision was quickly made to hold an online conference. So, with the technical help of Editmicro System we were able to have 117 people participate from 12 different countries! I learnt so much that year; drawing up online registration forms, providing information on recording presentations before the event, as we could not rely of overseas internet connections. For the actual conference, the planning committee were all together at the offices of Editmicro, and logistics for that included ordering food, sourcing sign language interpreters, ordering tee-shirts—a must for all conferences, and conference bags
Our final conference was a hybrid conference, held at the Artscape theatre complex in Cape Town, again with a great organizing committee! However, as with each conference, there were unforeseen situations and in this case was it not having access to funds, even though we did! Food had to be ordered beforehand which was the most stressful, as we only knew on the day how many people we needed to cater for! Many a spreadsheet was needed, for registration, types of disabilities, dietary needs, accommodation needs, flights to be booked. Meet and greet; shuttle transport, abstracts—their reviews and allocations. Many meetings were held and again Editmicro systems assisted us with the technology side as it was a virtual as well as an in-person conference. During the conference, as in the others, there was a lot of running around to do however this time I was in a 'Gogo' cart—a chair on wheels that you can steer, and so it was less taxing for me and more efficient for attending to the many 'needs' required
The aims and ambitions of AfriNEAD are of paramount importance on the—Need for Action of Disability—and although we have made a huge step on the research aspect on disability, what is seriously lacking is the action component!
And so, my wish for AfriNEAD, is that going forward and with every conference this dream will be realized.

References

Botha, M., & Ohajunwa, C. (2024). Seeing the human behind the research: Strengthening emerging African disability researchers. *African Journal of Disability, 13*, Article a1494. https://doi.org/10.4102/ajod.v13i0.1494

De Bont, A., Stoevelaar, H., & Bal, R. (2007, 7 December). Databases as policy instruments. About extending networks as evidence-based policy. *MBC Health Serv. Res., 7,* 200.

Daar, A. S., Berndtson, K., Persad, D. L., & Singer, P. A. (2007, 3 December). How can developing countries harness biotechnology to improve health? *BMC Public Health, 7,* 346.

Friedman, S. R., Mateu-Gelabert, P., Curtis, R., Maslow, C., Bolyard, M., Sandoval, M., & Flom, P. L. (2007, June). Social capital or networks, negotiations and norms? Neighbourhood case study. *Am J Prev. Med., 32*(6 Suppl), S160–70.

Information drawn from AfriNEAD programs and reports for conferences on the following years: 2007, 2009, 2011, 2014, 2017, 2020 & 2023. www.sun.ac.za/AfriNEAD

Kachaje, R., Dube, K., MacLachlan, M., & Mji, G. (2014). The African network for evidence-to-action on disability: A role player in the realisation of the UNCRPD in Africa. *AJOD, 3*(2).

Kahonde, C. K., & Mji, G. (2024). Disability research in African network for evidence-to-action in disability affiliated countries: An upward trend. *African Journal of Disability, 13*(0), a1517. https://doi.org/10.4102/ajod.v13i0.1517

Kitchin, R. (2005). *Towards emancipatory and empowering disability research: Reflections on three participatory action research projects*. National University of Ireland Maynooth.

Lau, D. C. (2004). *Tran, Mencius* (revised). Penguin Classics.

Mji, G., Gcaza, S., Swartz, L., MacLachlan, M., & Hutton, B. (2011). An African way of networking around disability. *Disability & Society, 26*(3), 365–368. https://doi.org/10.1080/09687599.2011.560419

Mji, G., Maclachlan, M., Melling-Williams, N., & Gcaza, S. (2009). Realizing the rights of persons with disabilities in Africa: an introduction to a special issue. *Journal of Disability and Rehabilitation, 31*(1), 1–6

Mozunder, P., & Marathe, A. (2007, 10 October). Role of information networks in malaria survival. *Malaria Journal, 6,* 136.

Ned, L. Y., Dube, K., & Swartz, L. (2022). Challenges and opportunities of centring the African voice in disability research. *African Journal of Disability, 11*, Article a1089. https://doi.org/10.4102/ajod.v11i0.1089

Robinson, M. (2007). Speech at the First AfriNEAD conference (SSEAD). Stellenbosch South Africa.

Sefotho, M. M. (2021). Basotho ontology of disability: An afrocentric onto-epistemology. *Heliyon, 7*(3), 8. https://doi.org/10.1016/j.heliyon.2021.e06540

CHAPTER 6

The Contribution of AfriNEAD to Disability Research in Africa

Callista Kahonde, Gubela Mji, and Malcolm MacLachlan

6.1 Introduction

Various definitions of disability emphasize how society's lack of responsiveness to the needs of persons with disabilities constitutes their disability rather than the nature of their difficulties per se. Increasing evidence on disability has allowed us to highlight factors that may facilitate the participation and inclusion of persons with disabilities in mainstream society. AfriNEAD recognized the critical role of research evidence and the need to use the evidence to start interfacing with different stakeholders that are expected to facilitate both the process of the production of research

C. Kahonde · G. Mji (✉) · M. MacLachlan
Cape Town, South Africa
e-mail: gumji@sun.ac.za

C. Kahonde
e-mail: ckkahonde@sun.ac.za

M. MacLachlan
e-mail: mac.maclachlan@mu.ie

G. Mji (ed.), *Doing Disability Research in Africa*,
https://doi.org/10.1007/978-3-031-98549-2_6

evidence and implementation of research at ground level for the realization of rights of persons with disabilities. Critically, AfriNEAD saw academic researchers as just one type of stakeholder in the evidence-to-action process. Disability advocates; local, national and international civil society; service provider organizations and practitioners, and governments are equally important stakeholders, and in fact more critical for addressing the evidence-to-action gap.

The network therefore explicitly wanted to develop a multi-perspective and interdisciplinary approach to addressing problems facing persons with disabilities in the African region. To our knowledge, as we embarked on this journey, this would be the only network, which sought to achieve such aims using research evidence as a prong to facilitate realization of the rights of persons with disabilities in the region. In this chapter, we will present the contribution of AfriNEAD to disability research since the inception of the network in 2007 and how this has impacted disability research in the region. Section. 6.2 highlight the pivotal role played by disability research in informing efforts to promote human rights and inclusive policies and practices in Africa.

6.2 Background

This background highlights the critical role of research in promoting disability rights and inclusion. Traditionally, persons with disabilities were viewed from a deficit perspective which ascribed all their experiences and the challenges they faced to the fact that they had bodily difficulties (Shakespeare, 2013). This medical model of disability worked together with the charity model where persons with disabilities had to rely on the goodwill of others to donate money and other resources they need to live (Retief & Letšosa, 2018). Research was also very much aligned with the medical model, whereby the focus was largely on understanding the disabilities and their causes and not the society or social barriers in which persons with disabilities live (Oliver, 1990). Persons with disabilities would rarely have a say in this kind of research that used them as models for experimentation (Phiri, 2014).

With the advent of the social model and human rights approaches to disability, which highlight the role that society plays in disabling people, came the discipline of disability studies (Davis, 2016). Disability studies is an interdisciplinary field that explores disability with a critical lens considering the cultural, political, social dimensions contributing to the experience of disability. It moves away from the traditional medical, charity and moral perspectives of disabilities to accentuating equality, justice, inclusion and human rights for persons with disabilities. Within this emancipatory lens, the focus of research has now moved to seeking understanding of daily lives of persons with disabilities and looking at the evidence with a critical perspective that questions why they are oppressed, marginalized and stigmatized. Persons with disabilities are now being given a more prominent voice in research, not only as research participants but as partners and co-researchers who help to shape the process of research and the implementation of the research findings. The research has many contributions ranging from understanding unique challenges faced by persons with disabilities in a largely ableist world and seeking solutions to these challenges, informing policy, advocacy and evidence-based practices in all areas like education, health, employment, family life and other major life areas. The research also contributes to developing accessible spaces and technologies, increasing disability awareness, reducing stigma and encouraging a common language for collaborations.

In Africa, disability prevalence is high but research that seeks to understand the reality of persons with disabilities is still scarce. Without relevant and grounded research, efforts to build inclusive societies may not address the things that matter most to persons with disabilities. Governments and other stakeholders may continue to perpetuate the oppressive systems and approaches while thinking they are doing the right thing. AfriNEAD realized an opportunity to promote the contribution of persons with disabilities in research and its implementation using a platform that connects them with other relevant stakeholders as noted above, and along with the business sector and others. Through the different activities outlined in this chapter, AfriNEAD has and continues to fulfil its mission of translating research into evidence-based advocacy, policy, practice and products, particularly in the pan-African context. It is important to note that being a regional network in Africa, AfriNEAD also plays a role in questioning disability research methods and theories developed elsewhere and promoting research that is more context relevant and appropriate to address issues that impact persons with disabilities in Africa, across its varied contexts, cultures and resources.

Conducting research is only the initial step, however, what is more important is ensuring that research is translated to policy and practice that promotes inclusion, human rights and dignity for persons with disabilities as enshrined in the UNCRPD. This is the gap that AfriNEAD recognized and is endeavouring to address, through its rich mix of partnerships both across sectors and across the continent.

6.3 Motivation for Establishing AfriNEAD

The Division of Disability and Rehabilitation Studies at Stellenbosch (DDRS) during the early stages of development of AfriNEAD expressed concern on the danger of the research community simply accumulating research evidence without using it to address the ways in which society can become more responsive to, and more inclusive of, the rights and abilities of persons with disability. Such oversight would replicate the very circumstances that constitute the disabling environments that we are concerned about and aim to address. Hence the DDRS developed AfriNEAD with the aim of addressing the challenge of translating research into evidence-based advocacy, practice and policy—particularly in the pan-African context. This was done with the understanding that disability research evidence in Africa needs to be systematically addressed in a coherent and ongoing fashion, addressing issues as they evolve over time. In this way the Division, through AfriNEAD hoped to become a leading Pan-African facilitator of evidence-to-action in disability.

6.3.1 AfriNEAD Research Objectives and Activities

As stated in previous chapters, AfriNEAD was inaugurated in November 2007. Its earlier business plan had objectives that were focused on production of disability research in the region and facilitating the translation of research evidence into transformative policy and practice. The sections that follow present the research objectives set out by AfriNEAD at its inception. For each objective, we highlight the intended impact and what has been achieved over the years that AfriNEAD has been in existence.

6.3.1.1 Best Evidence-to-Action Practice Guidelines

When AfriNEAD was established, one of its main objectives was the establishment of Disability Research Country Working Groups (DRCWG) in African countries that are affiliated to AfriNEAD. The DRCWGs would be tasked with identifying action pathways and producing Best Evidence-to-Action Practice Guidelines which would be published on the AfriNEAD website. These DRCWGs took some years to pick up mainly due to lack of resources, but they now exist in the following ten countries affiliated with AfriNEAD: the Democratic Republic of Congo, Ethiopia, Ghana, Kenya, Malawi, South Africa, Tanzania, Uganda, Zambia and Zimbabwe. This initiative started to bear fruit in the 2020 AfriNEAD conference and was formally launched at the 2023 AfriNEAD Conference.

The DRCWGs, whose membership mimics the membership of the mother body, are tasked with packaging the evidence and recommendations from the conferences as relevant to their local contexts. They also identify areas where there are evidence gaps in their local contexts and engage stakeholders who are potential role players in advancing disability research and evidence-based policy implementation. The AfriNEAD secretariat provides regular ongoing support to the DRCWGs through virtual meetings with country representatives of the DRCWGs. This encourages contact and networking of the groups themselves and sharing of ideas. At triennial conferences, each DRCWG is given space to share the status of disability research in their country and engage in dialogue with conference delegates on ways to continue advancing disability research and advocating for effective implementation. The next step that AfriNEAD is working on is collating outputs from each DRCWG that will be published on its website to keep the network informed about activities in each country and to encourage peer learning. Some of the recent activities of the DRCWGs will be outlined in the next chapter.

6.3.1.2 READ for Africa

The network planned collaboration with member countries by providing a methodology for them to undertake a situational analysis that would allow them to profile their own situation regarding disabled people, the services available to them, the research being undertaken, the research needed and identification of facilitators and barriers for turning research into policy and practice action. Every three years countries would submit their 'state of our nation' analysis regarding disability for publication in an E-book edited by the DDRS, and available for downloading on the AfriNEAD website. This triennial publication would be titled *Research on Evidence to Action in Disability for Africa (READ for Africa)* and would be distinguished by year of publication (READ for Africa 2009, READ for Africa 2012, etc.). This would be an important advocacy document as well as a product of the network's activities.

The postgraduate students (master's and PhD) undertaking their studies in the DDRS would contribute to 'READ for Africa' by publishing some of their master's and PhD research projects addressing the needs of member countries in this resource. It was anticipated that each year up to four countries could be targeted by postgraduate student research: either undertaking initial exploratory research profiling member countries or updating prior research. Such a focus was deemed strategic to encourage network member countries to fund postgraduate students, to facilitate this initiative.

One case study is that of the African Policy on Disability and Development project (APODD) (MacLachlan et al., 2014). The project had lead researchers from Ireland and South African, co-lead researchers from the then African Decade for Persons with Disabilities (Now African Disability Alliance) and the Division of Disability and Rehabilitation Studies (DDRS) at Stellenbosch University, Stellenbosch, South Africa. Growth and development of this project started organically from grassroots with the Chair from the African Decade assisting to link with Disabled Peoples Organizations (DPOs) from Ethiopia, Sierra Leone, Uganda and Malawi to choose persons with disabilities to function as research assistants for the project and register for master's programs at the DDRS. The people who were facilitating the research process of this project as research assistants were two post-doctoral fellows from Zimbabwe and Malawi. When not busy with their research activities, these research assistants also assisted the DPOs with activities related to administration. By the end of the project everybody had benefited. Table 6.1 shows the project outcomes:

From 2023, AfriNEAD established a PhD community of practice, which is promising as an avenue to build disability research evidence by postgraduate students in Africa. The community of practice is open to all current and recent PhD graduates in Africa. It was launched at the 2023 conference, through a workshop facilitated by recent PhD graduates, and well-attended by current PhD students and recent graduates from all over Africa. A reflective paper on the workshop and way forward for the community of practice was published in the African Journal of Disability (Botha & Ohajunwa, 2024).

6.3.1.3 AfriNEAD Conferences

Another objective was that the DDRS would organize a conference focusing on a particular issue of interest to network members. Initially,

Table 6.1 Project outcomes for the APPOD project

Project outcomes for the APPOD project
Alignment of the research project with article 31 of the CRPD • The South African Co-PI was a person with disability • 75% of in country researchers were persons with disabilities • These researchers continue to advance the work done by DPOs by assisting in administrative duties for these DPOs • Three of these researchers registered and completed their master's study at Stellenbosch University, Stellenbosch, South Africa and two out of three master's graduates were persons with disabilities • Research produced reports and policy briefs on status of inclusion of persons with disabilities in discussions on poverty reduction strategies in Sierra Leone, Malawi, Uganda, and Ethiopia and policy briefs in this area for these countries (MacLachlan et al., 2014)

the conferences were to be held every two years, but a decision was made after the 2011 conference to hold them every three years. The conference would address how research evidence can be put into advocacy, policy and rehabilitation practice, identifying facilitators and barriers and drawing on perspectives of persons with disabilities, carers, clinicians, managers, NGO's, civil servants, civil society, research funders and politicians. These conferences would invite researchers and practitioners to present their work to policymakers and challenge them to think-through the steps necessary to realize the rights of persons with disabilities. This would produce a unique and stimulating collection of papers from each conference that would be published as a special issue of a peer-reviewed journal. With each conference having a distinct theme, the AfriNEAD conferences would seek to publish a series of special issues.

Since its inauguration in 2007, AfriNEAD has managed to table seven conferences. The first three conferences were tabled biennially and the four that followed were tabled triennially. As mentioned in the previous chapter, the presentations and discussions were guided by eight research areas that the network members established and refined over the years. In 2020 assistive technology was added to the research areas, giving a total of nine areas that have been specified in the previous chapter. The Articles of the United Nations Convention on the Rights of Persons with Disabilities (UNCRPD) (UN, 2006) were used to guide the establishment of these nine research areas pertinent to the African context. In this way, AfriNEAD is promoting research that advances domestication of the UNCRPD in Africa.

The conference outputs have been published in special issues in internationally recognized peer-reviewed journals. The 2007 and 2009 conference papers were published in Disability and Rehabilitation as a special issue and an overarching paper on the 2009 conference was published in the Disability and Society journal. From 2011, AfriNEAD has had its own journal, the African Journal of Disability (AJOD), in which subsequent special issues were published.

6.3.1.4 African Journal of Disability (AJOD)

Though the AJOD was not initially presented as one of the objectives for generating research evidence for AfriNEAD, it became apparent in the annual general meeting of 2009 that there is a need to establish a journal that will provide a platform for disability researchers in Africa and beyond to publish their work. The AJOD is the product of collaborative efforts of AfriNEAD, the DDRS and Centre for Disability Studies at Kwame Nkrumah University of Science and Technology (KNUST) in Ghana and was launched at the 3rd AfriNEAD conference in Zimbabwe in 2011 with first issue published in 2012 and yearly after this.

Focus and Scope

The AJOD, the official journal of, AfriNEAD, DDRS and CEDRES is published by AOSIS and introduce and discuss issues and experiences relating to and supporting the act of better understanding the interfaces between disability, poverty and practices of exclusion and marginalization. Its articles yield new insight into established human development practices, evaluate new educational techniques and disability research, examine current cultural and social discrimination and bring serious critical analysis to bear on problems shared across the African continent. Emphasis is on all aspects of disability particularity in the low- and middle-income countries in the African context. Below in Table 6.2 is the scope of the African Journal of Disability (AJOD):

Publication Fees

The Article Processing Charges (APC) for this journal is **ZAR1494.00 (excl. VAT**) per A4 output page in PDF format for 2024. The average length of an article in this journal is **10** pages. This APC is valid for the

Table 6.2 Scope of the African Journal of Disability (AJOD)

Aspects included in the AJOD
- disability studies as an emerging field of public health enquiry—inclusive education - disability-related stigma and discrimination—disability and postcolonial issues—globalization and cultural change in relation to disability—disability, diversity and intersections of identity—disability and the promotion of human development—the role of arts and media in relation to disability—rehabilitation, including vocational and community-based rehabilitation—community development and medical issues related to disability and poverty—legal, policy, human rights and advocacy issues related to disability - disability as part of global Sustainable Development Goals transformation agendas—environmental and climate related issues linked to disability

current calendar year and may be changed at any time at the sole discretion of the publisher. The submitting author is responsible for payment of the APC and must confirm, at the time of submission, that she/he will organize payment of the APC, should the article be accepted for publication. This responsibility may not be delegated to any third party unless agreed to by the publisher. The APC fees have a huge implication for disability researchers in the region as most researchers from the region struggle to pay these fees. The AJOD has made a huge contribution to publication in Africa, but this is constrained by the APCs for open-source publishing.

Progress of the Journal

The AJOD has continued to gain recognition and to expand its reach. All articles published in the journal are included in: *African Index Medicus; AGORA; Directory of Open Access Journals (DOAJ); EBSCO Host; GALE, CENGAGE Learning; GOALI; Hinari; Norwegian Register for Scientific Journals, Series and Publishers, Level 1; OARE; ProQuest; PubMed Central.* The journal is an important platform for disseminating ongoing disability research in Africa and every three years, publishing research presented at the AfriNEAD conferences. Following each conference, a special issue dedicated to the conference is published in the journal. The special issues include editorials summarizing the main research themes emanating from the conference and conference outcomes related to disability research evidence in Africa. The Journal is on an upward thread in fulfilling its mandate of serving as being a platform for literature on disability scholarship which might assists scholars to start discussing

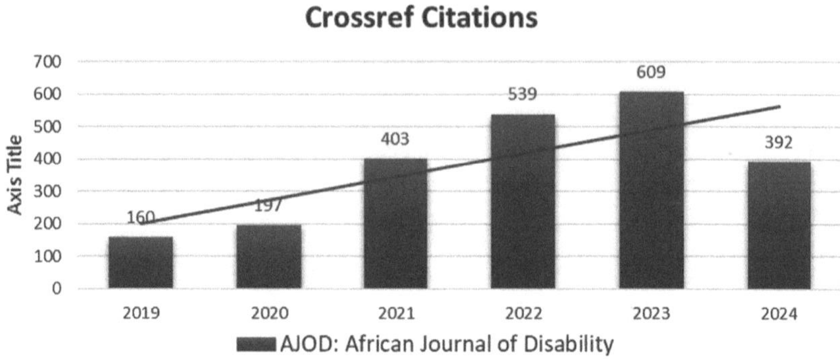

Fig. 6.1 Cross ref cited by statistics—data extracted at 15:00 18 June 2024 (AJOD, 2023)

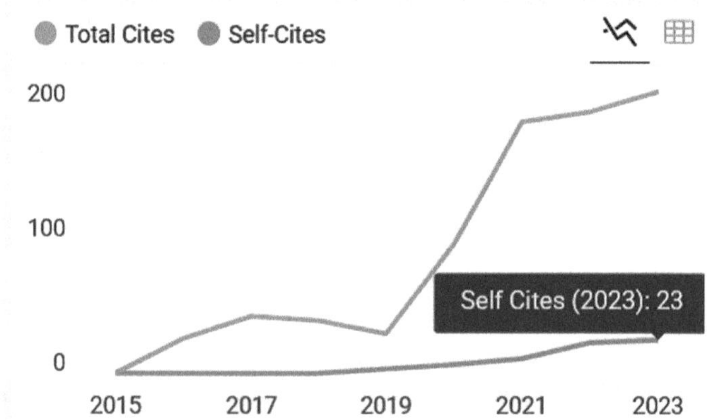

Fig. 6.2 Journal Self citation—data extracted at 14:00 9 July 2024 (AJOD, 2024)

what informs disability within the region and thereby starting to address the challenge of paucity regarding the disability theories that drive the disability debate within the region Below is Fig. 6.1 presenting citation of the publications from the AJOD from 2019 to 2023 (Fig. 6.2).

From these two figures one can see that there has been an increase in in the number of researchers using the AJOD. Indeed, there has been an upward trend in both the production of papers and the use of papers from the journal by researchers. The journal still poses a challenge for many researchers from the region due to authorship fees. The publisher offers authors with good publishable articles scholarship for their articles. South Africa continues to dominate publications for the journal because of reasons that will later be discussed.

To conclude this section, the efforts of AfriNEAD to have objectives that could assist the network to generate disability research evidence and to promote more research on disability in Africa have been clearly more successful in some areas than others. The AfriNEAD conferences have been tabled successfully as planned with outputs that generate the needed evidence for advocacy, policy development and implementation. The AJOD has also been successful in disseminating disability research on an ongoing basis and disseminating research evidence specifically from AfriNEAD conferences as special issues. The other objectives have been developing organically and will take some time to see their apparent outcome. The next sections of this chapter will cover: (a) Countries that have attended the seven AfriNEAD conferences; (b) number of papers that were presented for each thematic area; (c) discussion and (e) concluding statement.

6.4 Countries Attending the Six AfriNEAD Conferences

AfriNEAD conferences, since 2007 have been attended by delegates from thirty-nine countries, twenty-four of them being African countries. Each conference was attended by a few delegates from outside the Africa region who are interested in and supportive of the work of AfriNEAD. Some of them are researchers from other continents working on collaborative research in Africa with African researchers. The numbers of delegates attending the conference have increased over the years. Table 6.3 presents the countries represented at each conference and the respective number of delegates from each country.

Table 6.3 shows that countries that have hosted AfriNEAD conferences have a high number of participants. The total number of participants in AfriNEAD conferences from 2009 to 2023 (six conferences) is 928. There are 24 African countries and 15 international countries that have managed to send delegates to AfriNEAD conferences. From Africa, South Africa (224) has the highest number of participants attending

Table 6.3 Countries represented at AfriNEAD conferences and number of delegates from each country[1]

	Country	*2009*	*2011*	*2014*	*2017*	*2020*	*2023*	*Total*
1	Angola	0	2	0	0	0	0	2
2	Australia	0	1	0	0	1	0	2
3	Belgium	2	2	0	1	1	1	7
4	Botswana	3	5	1	3	2	1	15
5	Cameroon	0	0	1	1	0	5	7
6	Canada	0	0	1	0	1	2	4
7	Congo	0	0	0	0	1	0	1
8	DRC	0	0	0	0	6	2	8
9	Ethiopia	1	1	0	0	2	3	7
10	Finland	0	0	0	0	1	0	1
11	France	0	0	0	0	1	0	1
12	Germany	0	0	0	0	1	0	1
13	Ghana	8	2	2	144	2	13	171
14	Ireland	4	3	1	1	4	2	16
15	Kenya	4	2	0	0	0	3	9
16	Lesotho	0	5	0	0	1	0	6
17	Madagascar	0	0	1	0	0	0	1
18	Malawi	7	11	82	3	5	6	114
19	Mozambique	1	2	0	0	1	0	3
20	Mauritius	0	0	0	0	0	2	2
21	Namibia	4	8	0	1	4	2	19
22	Netherlands	4	1	0	0	0	0	5
23	Niger	0	0	0	0	0	6	6
24	Nigeria	4	4	0	0	1	2	11
25	Norway	5	4	0	3	4	9	21
26	Palestine	0	1	0	0	0	0	1
27	Rwanda	1	0	0	0	0	0	1
28	Sierra Leone	2	1	0	0	0	0	3
29	South Africa	64	36	24	22	85	93	224
30	Sudan	1	1	0	0	0	0	2
31	Swaziland	0	1	0	0	2	0	3
32	Sweden	0	0	0	0	1	0	1
33	Switzerland	0	0	0	0	3	0	3
34	Tanzania	0	0	0	0	13	8	21
35	Togo	0	0	0	0	1	0	1
36	UAE	0	0	0	0	1	0	1
37	Uganda	7	1	0	1	2	26	37
38	UK	5	2	1	2	4	8	22
39	USA	0	1	1	4	5	5	16

(continued)

[1] The green colour indicates the country that hosted the conference.

Table 6.3 (continued)

	Country	*2009*	*2011*	*2014*	*2017*	*2020*	*2023*	*Total*
40	**Zambia**	0	3	4	0	6	6	19
41	**Zimbabwe**	1	23	5	0	5	3	36
	TOTALS	128	123	124	186	167	208	928

AfriNEAD followed by Ghana (171) and Malawi (134). Other African countries that have a substantial number of attendees are Zimbabwe (36), Uganda (37), Tanzania (21), Namibia & Zambia (19) and Botswana (15). These numbers correspond largely with the trends of disability research published in AfriNEAD affiliated countries, as reported in a recent paper (Kahonde & Mji, 2024). Below under Table 6.4 are themes from the six AfriNEAD conferences, with abbreviation developed for Table 6.5 further below.

The number of papers presented at each conference fluctuates. As stated in chapter six, there were only six thematic areas for the conference in 2009, which were further refined to eight thematic areas for the conference in 2011, and with no papers for the thematic area on land/water, food and sanitation. This thematic area was later dropped due to lack of interest. In 2020 the thematic area on assistive devices was included and research evidence and utilization were presented in plenary as conference attendees felt that a bigger audience needed to hear presentations on this thematic area, and this was brought back to be presented with other

Table 6.4 Abbreviations for themes that were presented at the six AfriNEAD conferences

Abbreviations for themes that were presented at the six AfriNEAD conferences
1. Development process in Africa = DPA
2. Education = EDUC
3. Health & HIV and AIDs = H&HA
4. Holistic wellness = HW
5. Land/water and sanitation = LWS
6. Research Evidence = RE
7. Children and Youth = CY
8. Economic empowerment = EC
9. Systems of Community Based Rehabilitation = SCBR
10. Assistive Devices = AD

Table 6.5 Number of papers presented under each thematic area at the six conferences

	DPA	*EDUC*	*H&HV*	*HW*	*LWS*	*RE*	*CY*	*EC*	*SCBR*	*AD*
2009	11	9	18	3	2	15	0	0	0	0
2011	9	12	8	5	0	10	7	6	0	0
2014	11	13	10	11	0	12	10	11	11	0
2017	7	20	18	9	0	11	9	2	6	0
2020	5	6	4	7	0	0	6	6	6	8
2023	9	9	10	6	0	10	9	8	10	12
Total	52	69	68	41	2	58	41	33	33	20

thematic areas at the 2023 conference as sufficient papers were submitted to warrant this move.

6.5 Discussion and Recommendations

The intention of the network was that it will host two conferences in South Africa (SA) and then move to other African countries to host three conferences. Subsequently, it would return and host two further conferences in SA. The cycle would then be repeated. Countries that have hosted AfriNEAD conferences seem to have a substantial number of people who have attended the AfriNEAD conferences (South Africa, Zimbabwe, Malawi and Ghana). The network might need to rethink its strategy of hosting conferences to ensure that more conferences are hosted outside South Africa to improve the knowledge about the network and to ensure that other African countries are also engaged in the production of research evidence. The hosting of an AfriNEAD conference in a new country can be an important step in increasing awareness of and engagement with disability research.

Over and above the number of times AfriNEAD conferences have been hosted in South Africa, the country has the advantage of having three Universities offering disability studies courses (Universities of Cape Town, Stellenbosch and Pretoria). It is easy for academic staff from these universities, which tend to have resources to secure funding, to attend conferences. One can see that even when conferences were not hosted in South Africa, researchers from these units were able to attend AfriNEAD conferences as they were supported by their academic institutions. Availability of these disability studies units also makes the production of research evidence centralize around South Africa. If AfriNEAD is to achieve its vision of being the African network for evidence to action, it needs to ensure the participation of other countries in the production of research evidence.

It is also important to note that the countries that initially bid to host the conferences were countries that already have their academic institutions involved in disability studies and research. AfriNEAD supported Kwame Nkrumah University of Science and Technology (KNUST), Kumasi, Ghana, to develop academic programs in disability studies. At the time of writing the book, the next cohort of countries that have bid to host the 8th AfriNEAD conference in 2026 (Kenya, Ethiopia and Tanzania), these countries are already engaged in DRCWGs round tables for production of disability research evidence in their own countries. It would be encouraging to see that the country that is selected to host the conference is further supported to develop disability studies in the way that AfriNEAD did for KNUST.

AfriNEAD conferences are used by the network to advocate for disability research during the preparation for the conference and during the conference. For KNUST, the 5th AfriNEAD conference in 2017 offered the university an opportunity to organize the conference with College of Health Sciences of KNUST, since the event coincided with the college's 7th Biennial Scientific Conference. This occasion presented an opportunity to introduce AfriNEAD and disability research to every member of the college at KNUST which further advanced the dialogue that was needed between persons with disabilities, Disability Researchers and other professionals in KNUST.

AfriNEAD researchers also use the AfriNEAD conferences as a platform for dissemination of research outcomes. To facilitate this, researchers based in African countries are assisted with funding to attend AfriNEAD conferences, as we earlier saw, with projects such as African Policy on Disability and Development (APPOD) and the Equitable Projects. These were able to draw researchers from countries such as Namibia, Sudan, Sierra Leone, Uganda, Malawi, Ethiopia and recently Niger and Ghana, to attend AfriNEAD conferences.

There are 25 African countries and 16 international countries that have managed to send delegates to AfriNEAD conferences as shown in Table 6.3. It was also noted that some international countries sent substantial numbers of participants: UK (22), Norway (21), Ireland and USA (16). Some of these people are lead researchers of different disability projects conducted within the region. The UNCRPD article 32 puts emphasis on international cooperation for the support of persons with disabilities in low-income countries that are still struggling. One hopes that the next step with these researchers would be translation of this research evidence into action, as persons with disabilities within the region are tired of describing what they already know, what would be important to see how this research evidence is translated into action. This suggests that networks such as AfriNEAD should advocate to development of research agencies internationally to fund research through to its implementation, and associated evaluation, rather than only funding the earlier "discover" stages.

The lack of stability in AfriNEAD research themes seems to have contributed to fluctuation of the number of research papers presented in each conference. The addition of the theme on assistive devices in 2020 came as a follow-up from the intentions of the WHO Global Cooperation on Assistive Technology (GATE) project to motivate member countries to see this area as a priority, as it would be a challenge to achieve the inclusion of persons with disabilities without assistive devices.

The research themes that existed since 2009 seem to have an overall high number of papers presented except for the theme on land, water and sanitation. AfriNEAD opted to take this theme out of the call for papers for AfriNEAD conferences. With climate change being a topical issue in current times, it would be interesting to see whether researchers and disability practitioners who are engaged in this area of research are not struggling to find a platform to present research outcomes.

6.6 Chapter Conclusion

The chapter highlighted the different activities that AfriNEAD has engaged in to contribute to the disability research landscape in Africa. The network started with ambitious objectives and has managed to achieve some, and some which are still a work in progress. AfriNEAD prides itself in being the first network of its nature that brought together different stakeholders to promote disability research and implementation of research evidence into policy and practice in Africa. It also prides itself in ensuring that this is not a linear or one-way process, but rather a recursive, incremental and debated public process. It has provided

African researchers and other key stakeholders interested in disability with a platform to discuss, debate and disseminate their research and, through engaged dialogue, to enhance the impact of this research in respective countries. Looking at what the network has accomplished thus far, there is hope of increasing the disability research outputs in Africa through the influence of AfriNEAD. The establishment of DRCWGs in AfriNEAD affiliated countries is a promising fruit of the network towards more country specific and relevant research evidence to facilitate disability inclusive policy and practice.

References

AJOD (2023). Annual Journal Oversight Committee report. AOSIS, Durbanville RSA.

AJOD (2024). Indexing report. African Journal of Disability. AOSIS Durbanville RSA. https://cloud.3dissue.com/213197/213318/254414/AJODvol12/index.html

Botha, M. & Ohajunwa, C., (2024). Seeing the human behind the research: Strengthening emerging African disability researchers, African Journal of Disability 13(0), a1494. https://doi.org/10.4102/AJOD.v13i0.1494

Davis, L. J. (2016). *The disability studies reader*. Routledge.

Kahonde, C. K., & Mji, G. (2024). Disability research in African Network for Evidence-to-Action in Disability affiliated countries. *African Journal of Disability, 13*, Article a1517. https://doi.org/10.4102/ajod.v13i0.1517

MacLachlan M, Mji G, Chataika T, Wazakili M, Dube AK., Mulumba M, Massah B, Wakene D, Kallon F, Maughan M. (2014). Facilitating Disability Inclusion in Poverty Reduction Processes: Group Consensus Perspectives from Disability Stakeholders in Uganda, Malawi, Ethiopia, and Sierra Leone Disability and the Global South, OPEN ACCESS Vol.1, No. 1, 107–127 ISSN 2050–7364 www.dgsjournal.org

Oliver, M. (1990). The Politics of Disablement. Macmillan Education.

Phiri, A.M. (2014). Building communities of trust: Challenges for disability, *African Journal of Disability* 3(2), Art. #77, 3 ages. https://doi.org/10.4102/ajod.v3i2.77Retief, M. & Letšosa, R., (2018), Models of disability: A brief overview, HTS Teologiese Studies/ Theological Studies 74(1), a4738. 10.4102/hts.v74i1.4738

Retief, M., & Letšosa, R. (2018). Models of Disability: A brief overview. *HTS Teologiese Studies/Theological Studies, 74*(1).

Shakespeare, T. (2013). *Disability rights and wrongs revisited* (2nd ed.). Routledge, Taylor & Francis Group.

United Nations, (2006). *Convention on the rights of persons with disabilities*, viewed 02 July 2024, from https://www.ohchr.org/en/instruments-mechanisms/ instruments/convention-rights-persons-disabilities.

CHAPTER 7

The Development of Disability Research Country Working Groups

Gubela Mji, Hillary Lane, Dagnachew Wakene, Nondwe Mlenzana, Rosemary Choma, Patrick Devlieger, and Victor Locoro

7.1 Introduction

A Disability Research Country Working Group (DRCWG) is a country-based Working Group of disability researchers collaborating with other stakeholders in their home country (persons with disabilities, disability researchers and practitioners, government, business and civil society) (Kahonde & Mji, 2024). Wakene, 2011 emphasizes the importance of including researchers/academics with lived experience of disabilities who can assist in adopting the AfriNEAD concept locally to establish the state

G. Mji (✉) · H. Lane · D. Wakene · N. Mlenzana · R. Choma · P. Devlieger · V. Locoro
Cape Town, South Africa
e-mail: gumji@sun.ac.za

H. Lane
e-mail: hillarylane@outlook.com

D. Wakene
e-mail: dbwakene@gmail.com

G. Mji (ed.), *Doing Disability Research in Africa*,
https://doi.org/10.1007/978-3-031-98549-2_7

of disability issues in their country and identify areas that need intervention. Including persons with disabilities when developing DRCWG is further supported by Ned et al. (2022) in their paper which highlights the need of centring the African voice of persons with disabilities when conducting disability research.

Chapter 3, section three of this book, highlights the need for AfriNEAD's research and approaches to be driven and supported by ethics and emancipatory research and this should filter down to grass roots level and guide disability research (Kitchin, 2005). It is hoped and encouraged then that the scope of practice of DRCWGs about disability research is underpinned by good ethical principles and concepts (Strnadová et al., 2022; Tilley et al., 2021). By using good ethical principles and concepts, this will ensure that persons with disabilities are leading the dialogue in disability research thereby following the disability slogan: "nothing about us without us" (Koontz et al., 2022; Wakene, 2011). Persons with disabilities must be given space to decide what is important for them regarding the focus of in-country disability research (Botha & Ohajunwa, 2024). They are also encouraged and empowered to strengthen and support the voices of persons with disabilities who occupy different government departments (AfriNEAD conference program, 2023). Different countries are at different levels in terms of capacity; therefore, it is imperative to understand the environment and the capacity-building needs of persons with disabilities if the goal is that they should play their rightful position of leading the debates in disability research production (Botha & Ohajunwa, 2024).

AfriNEAD's intention is to contribute yearly reports to the Research on Evidence-to-Action in Disability (READ) for Africa, which compiles country profiles of their own local situations regarding persons with disabilities, the services available to them, the research being conducted, the gaps in policy and legislations and areas needing investigation

---

N. Mlenzana
e-mail: nmlenzana@uwc.ac.za

R. Choma
e-mail: rosechomakash@gmail.com

P. Devlieger
e-mail: patrick.devlieger@kuleuven.be

V. Locoro
e-mail: vlocoro@gmail.com

and identify facilitators and barriers for implementing research evidence (Kachaje, 2014). In this chapter we will present in detail the intention of developing DRCWGs including some of the struggles this AfriNEAD strategy experienced and a case study of a success story (AfriNEAD Conference program, 2023).

7.2 Background

DRCWGs are tasked with developing in-country research evidence together with action pathways. The groups are essential platforms for dialogue and debates, which engender change processes with principles of participation, consensus building and joint decision-making within AfriNEAD (Kahonde & Mji, 2024). The approach allows sharing of ideas, reduced bias, increased risk taking, high commitment and improved communication and overall, improved and effective approaches to the needs and rights of persons with disabilities at country level (Ned et al., 2022). This enables AfriNEAD as a network to get a broader picture of the area of disability at continental level (Mji & Edusei, 2019). This grouping can also act on advisory capacity as a vanguard about issues of the correct terminology, practices and approaches as well as instruments to use for National in-country research, such as—but not limited to—national statistics, inclusive decision-making processes on domestic policies and laws, inclusion and participation of persons with disabilities in elections, amongst several other interventions (Ebuenyi et al., 2023; Sait, 2023). DRCWGs contribute to AfriNEAD research objectives that have been mentioned in previous chapters by:

A. Developing a roundtable of people consisting of how AfriNEAD created its stakeholder group whereby AfriNEAD invited persons with disabilities, academic researchers involved in Disability research, Government, Business and Civil Society in what is called, the DAGBC Consortium where disability research will be discussed and way forward developed. Secondly, once AfriNEAD developed the nine thematic areas for development of research evidence for AfriNEAD (see Chapter 3) it was hoped that the DRCWGs would also follow this format for developing their research evidence at national levels (Kahonde & Mji, 2024).

B. Engaging Research on Evidence to Action in Disability for Africa (READ) in targeting DRCWGs in the development of the 'state of our nation' as this would be developed by DRCWGs. Such a focus may also encourage network member countries to fund students into the postgraduate programmes, to facilitate this. This would help to add to the cost effectiveness of the overall activities of the Division of Disability and Rehabilitation Studies (DDRS) (Mji & Edusei, 2019).
C. The AfriNEAD conferences offered the DRCWGs a platform where the Chairperson of each group will prepare a report about the status of disability research in their own country. Once the nine research focus areas were established from the fifty articles of the United Nations Convention on the Rights of Persons with Disabilities (UNCRPD)—this became the framework for the presentation of the status of disability research in their own countries (Kahonde & Mji, 2024). In the next section the position of DRCWGs within the structure of AfriNEAD is explained, this is followed by the aim and objectives and ends with the structure of DRCWGs.

7.3 The Position of DRCWGs Within the Overall AfriNEAD Strategy

Establishment and strengthening of functional DRCWGs is crucial as an AfriNEAD vehicle to reach out to many disability researchers, researchers with disabilities, persons with disabilities and other sectors who may not have contact or membership with the main network. While these in-country DRCWGs have the potential of giving AfriNEAD membership an understanding of the status of disability research in their own countries, they also ensure continuity of the work of AfriNEAD as the DRCWGs partake in implementing resolutions of the triannual conferences in a more country specific way. Thus, the UNCRPD, which is the basis for the themes and commissions of the triannual conferences (see Chapter 5), gets more attention and implementation in the different countries (Kahonde & Mji, 2024). Below are the aims and objectives for developing DRCWGs:

7.3.1 *Aims and Objectives of DRCWGs*

The overall aim of a DRCWGs is to adopt the concept of AfriNEAD at a local (country) level and context. In a way, the DRCWG is a mini-AfriNEAD which is country specific (Mji & Edusei, 2019). Below are the objectives for developing the DRCWG in countries that are participating in AfriNEAD.

7.3.2 *Objectives*

- To build critical mass for in country disability research and buy-in of the AfriNEAD concept at country level.
- To identify the main role players in disability research within the country and form meaningful partnerships with these role players.
- To establish a complete picture of the state of the nation with regards to disability research and identify gaps and the way forward in addressing them.
- To prepare a yearly overview of country status for publishing in the READ for Africa and the African Journal of Disability (AJOD).
- To format disability in country research evidence using the nine thematic areas of AfriNEAD that are underpinned by the UNCRPD.
- To present the work and findings of the DRCWGs at the triannual conferences.
- To domesticate and implement the UNCRPD through in-country research and its implementation and addressing the practical functioning of the AfriNEAD Commissions through domestication of resolutions from the triannual conferences using the nine thematic areas of AfriNEAD to different stake holders in a country, e.g. DPOs, government, academic institutions business and civil society formations (Kachaje, 2014).

7.3.3 *Structure of a DRCWG*

Membership in a DRCWG mirrors the AfriNEAD membership. Members from the disability, academic, government, business and the civil sectors form a DRCWG. With the understanding that disability should be a concern for everyone (Botha & Ohajunwa, 2024), membership is open to any person and organizations from these sectors who are interested in disability transformation through facilitating context relevant research and its translation into policy and practice.

Each DRCWG should have a coordinator who ensures effective and efficient running of the activities of the DRCWG and oversees the delivery of its programmes and raising sufficient funding resources (Mji & Edusei, 2019).

7.3.4 *The Role of AfriNEAD as the Mother Body and Support Base for the DRCWG*

DRCWGs are expected to take ownership of their local in-country activities and can be self-sustained. Initially they will receive support from AfriNEAD Secretariat and later at an ad hoc basis whenever necessary, AfriNEAD will do the following:

- Assist with initial set up of the DRCWG through training and capacity building.
- Hold annual meetings with the coordinators to touch base and provide necessary support.
- Publication of research evidence gathered by the DRCWG in the READ for Africa and AJOD.
- Provide consultation services, especially with conceptual components of the DRCWG activities.
- Advise on fund-raising opportunities (Mji et al., 2009).

7.4 Steps to Follow for Initiating a DRCWG

As a follow-up to the decision at the 2009 AfriNEAD conference to start focusing on the collation of regional disability research evidence, it became critical to implement some of the research-related objectives of AfriNEAD for production of research evidence for the network. There was an urgent need to implement country-based working groups throughout the AfriNEAD network (Kachaje, 2014).

Due to issues of capacity, the DRCWG strategy was mainly addressed during conferences when many African countries would be attending the AfriNEAD conference (Kahonde & Mji, 2024). There was also a perception that AfriNEAD could initially start with the Southern Federation for the Disabled (SAFOD) linked countries, but this never really materialized. What gave a break to the DRCWGs was COVID-19 and its lock-down with the increased use of technology during this phase (AfriNEAD conference program, 2020).

In planned workshops, the goal was to clarify the terms of reference for the AfriNEAD Disability Research Country Working Groups (DRCWGs) with reference to the AfriNEAD aims and to facilitate the translation of existing and new research in the disability arena into meaningful evidence-based advocacy, practice, products and policy in a coherent and consistent fashion, to realize equal opportunities and human rights for persons with disabilities. In these Workshops the goal was to establish the responsibilities of the working group members and establish membership of the working groups for each member country attending the workshop. To start a DRCWG group in each country the following steps were required:

7.4.1 In-country Preparatory Steps in Developing a DRCWG

- AfriNEAD members from a particular country needed to select a coordinator for the DRCWG.
- This coordinator works with the AfriNEAD Secretariat in setting up the DRCWG.
- The coordinator should meet with people (DPOs, disability researchers and practitioners, NGOs, Government departments, Business entities and civil society) who might be interested in disability research.
- Share the idea of developing a DRCWG for disability research evidence for that country, with the identified interested partners.
- Start developing a reference group to support the DRCWG in that country.

Below are aspects for discussion during the first workshop.

7.4.1.1 An Overview on AfriNEAD Commissions Covering the Following

- The link of the UNCRPD in the production of AfriNEAD research evidence.
- The development of the AfriNEAD 9 commissions/research thematic areas.

- How the Commissions will function with reference to the AfriNEAD working groups.
- The role of AfriNEAD commission leaders and the Commission leaders per AfriNEAD Country Working Group.
- The functioning of the AfriNEAD Commissions.
- The role of AfriNEAD as the mother body.

7.4.2 Participation During AfriNEAD Conferences

During the AfriNEAD conference coordinators for DRCWG from each country to move around commissions to continue planning for their own country working group and link with other country coordinators to network and gain support.

7.4.3 Coordinate Research Evidence for the Next Tri-annual Conference

- After the conference, coordinators are expected to continue with yearly preparation of overview of country status for publishing in the READ for Africa in the AJOD and this includes identification of gaps in disability research from their own countries.
- The goal was for future design of AfriNEAD conferences to be centred on the work of the DRCWGs, whereby research that is presented at country level is presented at the AfriNEAD conference using the nine thematic research focus areas drawn from the CRPD, unlike the fragmented individual research that was presented in the past.
- It is envisaged that post the 2023 conference, the country hosting the AfriNEAD conference, will focus on the work done by the DRCWGs, presenting the status of disability research in the nine thematic areas of the UNCRPD.
- Countries affiliated to AfriNEAD would in their own countries have symposia to collate disability research internally with the aim of developing an in-country report regarding the status of disability research to be presented at the tri-annual AfriNEAD conference.

7.5 Present Status of Disability Research Country Working Groups (DRCWGs)

As earlier stated, it has been a challenge to develop DRCWGs although there were more than twenty African countries affiliated to AfriNEAD. However, this strategy managed to gain some oxygen during COVID-19 and lockdowns (see Chapter 5).

The virtual platform created managed to assist AfriNEAD to lobby seven countries to participate in the 6th AfriNEAD conference: Ghana, Malawi, Uganda, South Africa, Tanzania, Zimbabwe and the Democratic Republic of Congo (DRC)/Kinshasa. At this juncture, these seven countries did not use the UNCRPD commissions for their presentations and some struggled a lot from issues of connectivity on the day they were supposed to present the status of disability research in their own countries in the AfriNEAD conference.

Despite this, the conference was encouraged to see the participation of these countries in the conference and the DRC was fortunate to have the Minister of Social Affairs, in charge of people with disabilities and other vulnerable groups presenting in the conference. The participation of this group encouraged the AfriNEAD Secretariat to strengthen the development of these groups and to ensure their participation in the 7th AfriNEAD conference in 2023.

7.5.1 *The Process of Strengthening the Countries with the Goal of Presenting in the 7th AfriNEAD Conference—a Case Study of a Success Story*

After hosting the 6th AfriNEAD conference, the AfriNEAD Secretariat started bi-monthly virtual training workshops to assist the DRCWGs. All the countries (DRC, South Africa, Tanzania, Ghana, Uganda and Zimbabwe) that participated in the 2020 6th AfriNEAD conference participated in this group of DRCWGs (AfriNEAD Conference report, 2020). The groups were also joined by Kenya and Zambia, and later during the conference, Ethiopia also joined the workshops.

The focus of the workshops was on capacity building of the DRCWGs, focusing on the above information. We also included training on empowerment, the WHO, Global Cooperation on Assistive Technology (GATE) project (Ebuenyi, 2023) and the Washington Group on Disability Statistics (WG) (Moreno et al., 2022). Closer to hosting the 7th AfriNEAD conference in 2023, we focused on data that was available in their countries to ensure that they could respond to the nine AfriNEAD research areas (Kahonde & Mji, 2024). We were also assisted by the South African Irish Embassy to ensure that these delegates could attend the conference in person and present a synopsis of disability research in their countries.

On the last day of the conference, the coordinators of three of the countries (Kenya, Tanzania and Ethiopia) entered the bid process to host the AfriNEAD conference in 2026. These ten countries also attended a presentation by Dr Charlotte McClain-Nhlapo (instead of the scheduled address which was to take place on Sunday 3 December). This was done to shorten a long conference. Thereafter, a consolidation workshop on "Disability Research Country Working Groups" was held and which created a vibrant discussion. On 3rd December—The International Day of Persons with Disabilities—was marked by a tour by the DRCWGs around the Cape Peninsula in the Western Cape Province in South Africa. The day was held in a celebratory mode. Table 7.1 is a summary of key points that emerged from their conference presentation:

2023 conference programme.

7.6 Summary Regarding the Presentation of Countries

- The ten countries (DRC, Ethiopia, Ghana, Kenya, South Africa, Tanzania, Uganda, Malawi, Zambia and Zimbabwe) that participated in the exercise of collating data form their countries and aligning it with the nine AfriNEAD thematic areas seem to have a good grasp of how to align the disability research evidence in their countries with the nine AfriNEAD thematic areas.
- Not every country could respond to the nine thematic areas due to the absence of research evidence in these areas in their countries.
- Most of the countries have their research evidence funded by external agents, and this raised the issue of sustainability and ability to translate research evidence into action.
- It appears that countries with research evidence were struggling to hold their governments accountable in translating research evidence into action that will assist in improving the lives of persons with disabilities.

Table 7.1 Summary of key points that emerged from DRCWs synopsis

Congo (DRCNEAD): 1. No structured research networks related to disability. There are a few independent researchers who devote themselves in disability research. Intention to follow up and initiate these themes in our universities in collaboration with independent Congolese researchers 2. Assistive technology, in the DRC, precisely in Kinshasa, there is a structure called rehabilitation centre for the physically handicapped (CRHP) 3. A social assistance service is also available for people requiring support services 4. There is also an optical, musculoskeletal and orthopaedic centre that offers orthopaedic equipment, and optical service. Equipment manufactured by this centre is expensive that most disabled people cannot afford 5. Studies on spiritualties related to people with disabilities are unfortunately not impacted especially on the lives of children with disabilities qualified as sorcerers in several places of the country, especially in rural areas	South African (SANEAD): 1. South Africa is in a unique position with disability studies units in the Western Cape (2), & Gauteng 2. SANEAD has information and could respond easily to all the nine thematic areas 3. This research is happening in silos with minimal collaboration 4. There is a need for interdisciplinary studies, which will assist in seeing disability as an intersectional agenda 5. There might be a need to create a repository of disability data and make it available to anyone who wants to do research and AfriNEAD could play this coordination role of disability research

(continued)

Table 7.1 (continued)

Ethiopia (EthioNEAD): 1. Started late in preparing for the 2023 conference 2. Ethiopia has been involved in AfriNEAD since 2008 through a research project called African Policy on Disability and Development (APODD) 3. There is a strong sense in AfriNEAD that Ethiopia should be a role player in the DRCWGs with the goal of establishing an AfriNEAD office with the African Union (AU) in the Ministry of Social Affairs 4. The representative for Ethiopia, an alumnus of the master's Programme through the abovementioned APODD research project. 5. EthioNEAD has entered the bid process to host the 8th AfriNEAD conference in 2026	Tanzania (TanzaNEAD): 1. Country Population: 62 ml. people; (HCP, 2022), 11.2% equivalent to 5.2 million are persons with disabilities 2. Achievements amongst others are: Endorsed the constitution, bank account, website and email system, Board of directors increased from 20 to 40 members 3. Strong desire from TanzaNEAD for a disability stand-alone census for persons with disabilities addressing specific needs are hard to capture from the general national house and population census 4. TanzaNEAD responded to the nine thematic areas with research evidence of 144 articles, research mainly from NGOs funded with external funding 5. TanzaNEAD, has entered the bid process to host the 8th AfriNEAD conference in 2026

(continued)

Table 7.1 (continued)

Ghana (GhaNEAD):	**Uganda (UgaNEAD):**
1. GhaNEAD responded with some information for the nine thematic areas 2. Research revealed that PWDs enjoyed limited support from government agencies and communities when donor funding for community-based rehabilitation (CBR) projects got to the end 3. The Government could also enact policies to exempt PWDs from paying premium on National Health Insurance Scheme (NHIS) 4. The 3% of the District Assembly Common fund meant to be released at quarterly for PWDs either unduly delayed or were not released at all 5. There is a need for more advocacy to motivate Government of Ghana to subsidize the cost of assistive devices. More advocacy to motivate Government to implement research output and policies about PWDs to practice, i.e. translating research evidence to action	1. Despite the strong disability activism that the country has had since the 1990s, research on disability is limited 2. Studies undertaken from early childhood to tertiary (13 studies); Economic empowerment (eight studies) and Development process in Africa (0) 3. Research is mainly funded by Donor & NGO 74% 4. Despite the good laws and policies on disability in the country; implementation is poor 5. Need to promote research on disability and use of findings to inform policy and programming in the country

(continued)

Table 7.1 (continued)

Kenya (KeNEAD): 1. There are 47 round tables across all the counties to help us receive inputs that are contextually relevant 2. Aim to launch a national secretariat to help DRCWG members reach grassroots 3. The DRCWG has an office comprised of the national coordinator, a secretary from the government, CSO's, academia, faith-based groups and a disability mainstream 4. There is high amount of independent research from development partners, however very little help government craft programs for PWDs 5. KeNEAD, has entered the bid process to host the 8th AfriNEAD conference in 2026	**Zambia (ZAMNEAD)** 1. There is some evidence on the 9 thematic areas produced by Government/International Organisations/NGOs 2. Disability Policy not yet fully implemented due to Government's failure to allocate priority and adequate budget 3. There is absence of awareness campaigns on the availability of the persons with disabilities (PWD) Act No. 6 of 2012 and its content 4. Compliance to the Persons with Disability Act is almost insignificant due to the absence of; monitoring and enforcement of penalties to non-compliance 5. Non-compliance of government institutions gives a very big opportunity for the private sector and NGOs not to comply
Malawi (MalaNEAD): 1. The Centre for Social Research has collaborated with many research institutions over the last two decades. Most notably is SINTEF in Norway and Trinity College in Dublin and Maynooth University in Ireland 3. We have disseminated the results from these studies widely including to policymakers in Malawi and the evidence has been used to inform policy and programming 4. There is available disability data that could be aligned to the 9 AfriNEAD thematic areas 4. This data is housed in different institutions, e.g. National Statistical Office, is located and where University of Malawi is located - there might be a need to create a repository of disability data and make it available to anyone who wants to do research 5. There is a need to strengthen our AfriNEAD country working group	**Zimbabwe (ZimNEAD):** 1. Persons with disabilities occupying strategic positions: Judge; Zimbabwe Election Commissioner, Chief Director in government ministries 2. Organizations of Persons with Disabilities are now getting more involved in research as it is now becoming funders' requirement to engage them 3. There was the adoption of the National Disability Policy in 2021 4. There is available of data on the nine thematic areas 5. Research institutions are still yet to make a deliberate effort to fund disability research

- There is a need to first strengthen the DRCWGs in each country to play the vanguard role of using disability research to hold governments accountable to persons with disabilities and there is a need to develop this roundtable in countries that do not have DRCWGs (Kachaje et al., 2014; Kahonde & Mji, 2024).

7.7 Chapter Conclusion

The goal of establishing working groups in countries affiliated to AfriNEAD was to ensure that AfriNEAD develops a grass root understanding of the status of disability from these countries (Mji et al., 2009). The AfriNEAD conferences offered the DRCWGs a platform where the chairperson/coordinator of each group will prepare a report about the status of disability research in their own countries (Mji & Edusei, 2019). Once the nine research focus areas were established from the fifty articles of the UNCRPD—this became the framework for the presentation of the status of disability research in their own countries. The DRCWGs also act as a vehicle to facilitate the translation of disability research into policy and practice. It is a strategy to ensure that, at country level, research on disability is translated into meaningful evidence-based advocacy, practice, products and policy to ensure equal opportunities and realization of human rights for persons with disabilities (Mji & Edusei, 2019). In a way, the DRCWGs are a mini-AfriNEAD which is country specific.

This grouping can also act in an advisory capacity as a vanguard about issues of the correct terminology and approaches as well as instruments to use for National statistics and ensuring inclusion and participation of persons with disabilities in elections.

References

AfriNEAD conference programs: 2020 & 2023. www.sun.ac.za/AfriNEAD

Botha, M., & Ohajunwa, C. (2024). Seeing the human behind the research: Strengthening emerging African disability researchers. *African Journal of Disability, 13*, Article a1494. https://doi.org/10.4102/ajod.v13i0.1494

Ebuenyi, I. D., Smith, E. M., Jamali, M. Z., Munthali, A., & MacLachlan, M. (2023). The IDEAL PROCESS for developing assistive technology policy. *Assistive Technology, 36*(3), 224–231. https://doi.org/10.1080/10400435.2023.2254359

Kachaje, R., Dube, K., MacLachlan, M., & Mji, G. (2014). The African network for evidence-to-action on disability: A role player in the realisation of the UNCRPD in Africa. *AJOD, 3*(2).

Kahonde, C., & Mji, G. (2024). Disability research in AfriNEAD affiliated countries: An upward trend. *African Journal of Disability.*

Koontz, A., Duvall, J., Johnson, R., Reissman, T., & Smith, E. (2022). "Nothing about us without us:" Engaging at users in at research. *Assistive Technology, 34*(5), 499–500. https://doi.org/10.1080/10400435.2022.2117524

Kitchin, R. (2005). *Towards Emancipatory and Empowering Disability Research: Reflections on Three Participatory Action Research Projects*. National University of Ireland Maynooth.

Mji, G., MacLachlan, M., Melling-Williams, N., & Gcaza, S. (2009). Realising the rights of disabled people in Africa: An introduction to the special issue. *Disability and Rehabilitation, 31*(1), 1–6.

Mji, G., & Edusei, A. (2019). *An Introduction to a Special Issue on the Role of Assistive Technology in Social Inclusion of Persons with Disabilities in Africa: Outcome of the Fifth African Network for Evidence-to-Action in Disability Conference Afr J Disabil.* https://doi.org/10.4102/ajod.v8i0.681

Moreno, J. D., Bennett, L. H. V., & Ferrite, S. (2022) The use of the Washington group on disability statistics questionnaires to identify hearing disability: A systematic review. *Codas. 12;34*(2), e20200328. https://doi.org/10.1590/2317-1782/20212020328. PMID: 35043863; PMCID: PMC9769417.

Ned, L. Y., Dube, K., & Swartz, L. (2022). Challenges and opportunities of centring the African voice in disability research. *African Journal of Disability, 11*, Article a1089. https://doi.org/10.4102/ajod.v11i0.1089

Strnadová, I., Dowse, L., & Garcia-Lee, B. (2022). *Doing research inclusively: Co-production inaction*, Disability Innovation Institute, UNSW, Sydney.

Tilley, E., Strnadová, I., Ledger, S., Walmsley, J., Loblinzk, J., Christian, P. A., et al. (2021). "Working together is like a partnership of entangled knowledge" Exploring the sensitivities of doing participatory data analysis with people with learning disabilities. *International Journal of Social Research Methodology, 24*(5), 567–579. https://doi.org/10.1080/13645579.2020.1857970

Wakene, G. B. (2011). The role of disability rights movements in the Ethiopian development Agenda. (Masters thesis). University of Stellenbosch.

Sait, W. (2023). An exploration of disability experiences and responses of disabled persons and their families within Muslim culture of the community of Strand, South Africa. PhD thesis. Stellenbosch University, South Africa.

CHAPTER 8

African Perspective on Disability

Gubela Mji, Nomvo Dwadwa-Henda, and Chioma Ohajunwa

8.1 Introduction

The African Network for Evidence to Action in Disability (AfriNEAD) aimed to use research evidence as a prong for the realization of rights of persons with disabilities. The goal of AfriNEAD was to use disability research evidence at policy and practice interphase to ensure that services are responsive to the needs of persons with disabilities. Initially disability theory and research evidence were mainly dominated by a group of British sociologists (Barnes, 1992; Oliver, 1992). In the African region, the lens utilized for the exploration of disability, as a concept, and the lived experiences of persons with disabilities, have emanated from the Global North until now when disability academic scholars from the Global South

G. Mji (✉) · N. Dwadwa-Henda · C. Ohajunwa
Cape Town, South Africa
e-mail: gumji@sun.ac.za

N. Dwadwa-Henda
e-mail: nhenda@sun.ac.za

C. Ohajunwa
e-mail: chioma@sun.ac.za

G. Mji (ed.), *Doing Disability Research in Africa*,
https://doi.org/10.1007/978-3-031-98549-2_8

are emerging. This thinking and conceptualization of disability from the Global North is constructed through social processes and philosophical influences that inform and position groups within society, instituting a hierarchical individual approach to people and groups. These approaches might be in contradiction with the collective approach that is mainly used by Africans. Disability studies is a new enquiry in African academic institutions. These studies tend to lean more on Global North in conceptualizing and theorizing disability for their programs. There is a need to start initiatives that are led by African researchers and persons with disabilities to dialogue on an African thinking and conceptualization of disability in Global South.

8.1.1 Background

There is paucity on information on African thinking and conceptualization of disability in African academic institutions. Available literature tends to present African response to persons with disabilities heavily skewed towards negativity and exclusion. Sefotho (2021) explains that indigenous ontologies have for many centuries endured epistemological subjugation from Euro-Western epistemologies. He further expands that these indigenous ontologies within the field of disability, encountered "oppressive discourses of disability" which side-lined indigenous knowledge systems. Chikane (2012), quoting Mbeki, points to different groups of people that have entered the African continent and asserts that these new entries, have somehow continued to shape and evolve both the knowledges and beingness of an African person, including how Africans define and respond to disability (Mji, 2019). Sefotho (2021) points to the fact that contrary to a heavy skew towards negativity ascribed to disability, the Basotho ontology brings about a positive disposition that promotes inclusion of children with disabilities in society.

Disability studies, like race, gender and sexuality, has been absent in African academic institutions. These identity categories and other forms of our identity are closely interwoven and intersect with each other on many levels that they end up contributing to social inequality and oppression that are felt in multiple forms of discrimination (Ned, 2015). It is also well documented that academic exclusion is a big issue for persons with disabilities from primary to higher education institutions. This implies that the initial conceptualization of disability research in African academic institutions will be conducted mainly by non-disabled people. It is easy for these scholars to use available information from the Global North without directly engaging persons with disabilities on their lived experience.

The South African disability rights movement in the 1990s adopted the saying, “Nothing About Us Without Us” and this became the clarion call of activists organizing to overcome systemic oppression and empower persons with disabilities to take control over decisions affecting their lives. This call aims to achieve the full participation and equalization of opportunities for, by and with persons with disabilities. AfriNEAD tends to align itself with this clarion call, seeing persons with disabilities being central and playing multiple roles in the production of disability research: participants, lead researchers and others.

There is an urgent need to develop an African disability thinking and conceptualization in African academic institutions. Central to the development of this African thinking about disability is the participation of persons with disabilities to destabilize power-relations within the research agenda and processes. Kitchin (2005) asserts that disability research should be wrestled free from academic researchers who are still using traditional research methodologies and, as such, call for the adoption of research strategies that are both emancipatory (seeking ‘positive’ societal change) and empowering (seeking ‘positive’ individual change through participation). The following sections are covered in this chapter: African disability perspective; disability and African spirituality is outlined followed by a case study of the AmaBomvane perspective on disability and rituals, the need to re-conceptualizing perspectives about African disability thinking and the chapter finishes with chapter conclusion.

8.2 African Perspective on Disability

African perspectives on disability often diverge from Western representations, offering views rooted in communal, spiritual and cultural values. In her work on spirituality, Ohajunwa (2019) highlights how disability in many African contexts is interpreted through integration of spiritual and cultural beliefs, making its management more holistic and tied to the moral, spiritual and community fabric of life. These interpretations often inform the ways in which families, including kinship networks, respond to people with disabilities. In many situations, the care and inclusion of persons with disabilities takes the form of a collective responsibility. However, with the domination of disability conceptualization and heavy reliance on Global North (Grech, 2015; Meekosha, 2011), many contextual factors surrounding disability become missed opportunities, impacting interpretations of this concept and development of attitudes towards persons with disabilities. A similar sentiment is expressed in literature that conceptualizing of disability in the hands of Global North is saturated with misconceptions about Africa, resulting in the exclusion of African indigenous knowledge systems (Bezzina, 2018; Bradbury-Jones et al., 2018; Comaroff & Comaroff, 2012). In her work on indigenous research, Mji (2019) also decries the weakening of the indigenous peoples' knowledges by the colonisers, resulting in spiritual disruptions, which later moved people to action to ensure that their heritage does not die. Today, the perceptions of disability are influenced by ***'ableism'*** "a system that places value on people's bodies and minds based on societally constructed ideas of normality, deeply rooted in anti-Blackness, eugenics, misogyny, colonialism, imperialism, and capitalism" (Lewis, 2020, p. 1). These imperial ideologies and colonial relations of knowledge production which are fostered upon Africa continually characterize and shape the academic space, need dismantling (Grange, 2009) to provide a nuanced Afrocentric approach that drives the African disability agenda.

The common narrative that Western knowledges is grounded in science while Indigenous knowledges are based on oral tradition (Bruchac, 2020) may have an impact on the adoption of Western conceptualization of disability as universal. Research on disability in most parts of Africa, with South Africa included, is mostly conceptualized along cultural beliefs, attitudes and stigma and religious perspectives of Western origins (Inguanzo, 2017; Nyangweso, 2018). In most cases, conceptualizations of disability research in Africa portray disability as a liability. For example, research conducted in Southern Africa shows that persons with disabilities are excluded in social and economic developmental initiatives and are not even considered in policy formulation and implementation for they are seen as incapable (Dube & Charowa, 2005; Eide et al., 2014; Tigere & Moyo, 2022). Culture is used to discriminate against people with disabilities and the negative attitudes seem to be rooted in traditional practices (Rohwerder, 2018). However, there is leniency towards dominant Western knowledges while African traditional knowledge is still struggling to occupy centre stage. When such accommodation is made, it is important to consider that indigenous people were systematically excluded from taking charge of their own history (Smith, 2012). Redress can only occur through decoloniality of disability theories. Indigenous research on disability conducted in Africa, also needs scrutiny to ensure that it does not fall short of acknowledging the hard work done by scholars in the southern hemisphere. Given the above, and, while not attempting to present a glorified African account of disability, it is imperative to note that there are various discourses that can inform African thinking and concepts on disability.

The following section will refer to some discourses that inform African thinking and concepts of disability, i.e. (i) Ubuntu; (ii) Ancestor reverence; (iii) All people are equal and (iv) disability and spirituality.

8.2.1 Ubuntu Philosophy

In African contexts, the concept of *Ubuntu*—"I am because we are"—emphasizes the interconnectedness of people and the community's responsibility to support people with disabilities. The focus is often on communal wellbeing and shared responsibility for the care and inclusion of others. Drawing from a Southern African experience, we use the Basotho proverb that features *Ubuntu* towards a child with disability: 'Sehole ho' 'Ma-sona ha se lahloe' 'a child with a disability is never abandoned by the mother' (Leshota & Sefotho, 2020; Sefotho, 2021). It is a worldwide view that mothers care for their children, however, the difference in the story of the Basotho lies in their recognition of the existing bond between mother and child and utilizing that strength as a campaign to enhance protection of children with disabilities. The use of proverbs in the understanding of African thought and folklore has long been used in African society to generalize a community's experience which portrays the original situation (Kisanji, 1995). Proverbs have also been used in explaining complex social issues and simplifying them so that people grasp the concepts including disability (Lubinga, 2014). In the case of the Basotho, the proverb is embraced by the people because it touches on the hearts of parents, especially mothers, and promotes inclusion of persons with disabilities. The fact that it is in the language that people speak, people take ownership. In addition, the Basotho approach is deemed compassionate toward disability because it carries respect and permits others in the community to embrace a person with disability (Parsloe, 2015). The mother's resilience and compassion resonate with what Masasa et al. (2005) describes as caring families, regardless of whether the child has a disability.

8.2.2 Ancestor Reverence

Ancestor reverence is a way of understanding the world and not a religious system as Western thought assumes it to be. It pertains to the general belief that something of the dead person does not wholly disappear and is given substance by respecting those who have died (Mji, 2013). In this section, we draw from an indigenous Akan experience in Ghana where a mother decided to keep her daughter with disability, as a loving expression of Indigenous kinship, denying the 'mercy killing' that was recommended by hospital staff (Gyamfi, 2021). This situation attests to the diversity of African perspectives on disability, shaped by tradition, spirituality, collectivism and human dignity, which brings a balance in society. In the Ghanaian experience, the involvement of extended kin members, including the elders, signifies the importance of giving a good report to the ancestors should misfortune occur to the child. Reverence towards ancestors (Berg, 2003) which permeates this African experience, contains the tenets outlined in the Convention on the Rights of Persons with Disabilities (CRPD) (United Nations, 2006). This observation brings about a question: Are the philosophical foundations of the CRPD aligned with African discourses? This question is prompted by the realization that the African way of being and doing is as old as time immemorial.

8.2.3 All People Are Equal

In this section we draw from the indigenous Maasai peoples of Kenya, where disability is not a standard for classifying others. They believe all people are equal and recognize varying forms of impairments while their interaction with people is not related to their impairments (Talle, 2020). Similarly to the Classification of Functioning, Disability and Health (ICF) model (WHO, 2001), the Maasai only consider a person to have a disability when one is unable to perform daily work. When people with disabilities participate in community rituals, the chances of being acknowledged and even valued by others are increased, and so is acceptance (Stone-MacDonald & Butera, 2012). This finding is comparable to disability study findings of indigenous people in South Africa (Dwadwa-Henda, 2023). The Maasai value good moral standards that are uplifting to women such as fairness, equality and dignity, and which are put into practice by giving recognition to women with disabilities including their children by granting them entitlement to the inheritance of family property (Talle, 2020).

8.2.4 African Spirituality

African spirituality or the spirituality of the African is deeply holistic, embedded and connected with not only the inner being of the individual, but also the external environment surrounding the existence of the individual and how the individual interacts with that environment (Ohajunwa et al., 2021). African spirituality comprises a three-fold multidimensional *relationship* that includes humans, physical spaces and other lives that exist in our environment and the divinity. This is a foundational belief system. Therefore, the conception, understanding, presentation and expression of African spirituality are lived within the collective.

Historically, some scholars have questioned the existence of a spirituality that is 'purely African' arguing that external religious influences like Christianity, and then also Islam, have entered Africa and impacted the African ways of knowing (van Binsbergen, 2011 cited in Amanze, 2011). This argument of external influence has been put forward to marginalize the African understanding of spirituality. Amanze (2011) presents that even though the term 'African' is contested, he further agrees with James, (2015) and Wheeler et al. (2002), who hold that despite this contestation, spirituality is not 'set', 'ruled' or 'tenanted' by any one specific group, but the understanding and expression of spirituality is contextual and cultural. Hence African spirituality exists: a form and expression of spirituality that informs the being, doing and continuous becoming of the African through spiritual holistic relationships with humans, the physical environment and the divinity.

Spirituality encompasses practical actions (doing), and a sense or perception of 'knowing', (Chuengsatiansup, 2002; Ferrer, 2011) which speaks to the being and becoming of the person. Within the tenets of the African belief system, there is no separation of the being, doing and becoming, therefore the 'sensing' and the 'practical' go hand in hand, hence spirituality is positioned as a way of life and practised holistically (Chilisa, 2012; James, 2015). An example is the African spiritual philosophy of Ubuntu. The very tenet of Ubuntu enshrouds the being, doing and becoming (Sense and practicalities) (Ohajunwa et al., 2022). First within Ubuntu, we see that we do not exist alone. We have such an integral connection to the other (Humans, animals, physical environment, divinity) that we only exist in direct relation to the existence of the other, we recognize that we exist, because the other does. This is a spiritual tenet (The Being). Based on this understanding of a shared Beingness, we engage and transact (The doing) (Ohajunwa, 2019). We realize that in continuously engaging in respectful transactions with the other—human, animals, physical environment and divinity, we ourselves are also continuously becoming. The becoming is informed by both the practical and the spiritual, which enables us to keep transcending and connect to a higher egalitarianism (Ohajunwa, 2019).

Ohajunwa (2019) speaks on how colonization has influenced the spirit of Bomvane to go into hiding and when it attempts to emerge from hiding, it is no longer the original spirit of the Bomvane person but a spirit that is combined with some elements of the spirit of the colonizer. The often negative and invasive impositions of the western worldview of disability on African thought is a reality and has contributed to the ambivalent experiences of disability within various African contexts (Ohajunwa & Sefotho, 2024). Despite this ambivalence, this foundational, philosophical understanding of spirituality discussed here influences how many African communities engage with the concept of disability and persons with disabilities.

8.2.5 Case Study of AmaBomvane

AmaBomvane or the Bomvana, (as they are alternatively called) are people who strongly adhere to customs, traditions and ancestral reverence where spirituality forms part of family resilience. It is their traditional belief system that holds them together. Traditional beliefs, relationships, common interests, Ubuntu and social organization are all relational and thus constitute a system that is broadly defined as Indigenous or traditional knowledge. Commitment to this value system is believed to have beneficial impact on the entire collective as reflected in their indigenous worldview in Fig. 8.1. Life-cycle rituals are believed to secure a person and the community's wellbeing and afford people the ability to bounce back from negative experiences and traumas caused by disruptions in their cultural belief system (Dwadwa-Henda, 2023; Ohajunwa, 2019). Below in Fig. 8.1 is the indigenous worldview of AmaBomvane.

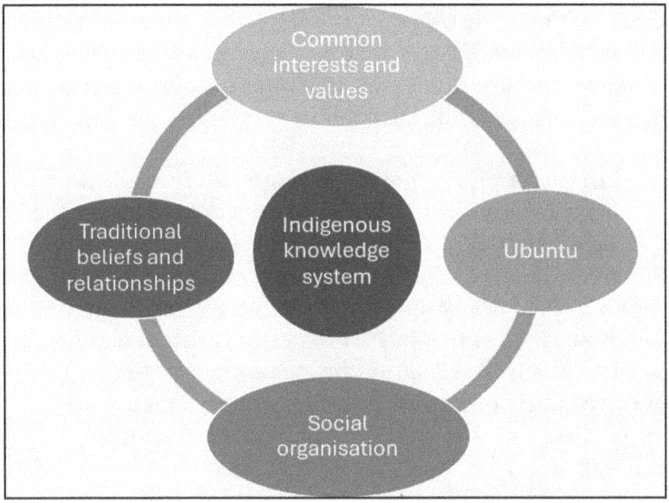

Fig. 8.1 Indigenous worldview of AmaBomvane (Dwadwa-Henda, 2023)

8.2.5.1 Social Organization

Life of AmaBomvane goes beyond the social unit of the extended family which occupies a homestead. In the homestead there is an agnate main male member who is linked to other clan members outside the homestead which now becomes a social structure. This social structure (comprising of clans) account to the Chief as the head of the community.

8.2.5.2 Rituals, Traditions, Relationships, and Common Interests

Because each family group is linked to a wider group, they share common ancestors, and common interests which bind them together. The relationship is characterized by a continuous process of mutual engagement, which emphasizes the coexistence of all beings regardless of physical or mental differences. These relational frameworks extend to people, land and spiritual world, valuing all contributions. The focus is on what people can offer rather than what they lack.

8.2.5.3 Ubuntu

Underlying all the above is the interdependence on one another, which is displayed by the Bomvana affection of their fellow man, and the respect bestowed throughout their engagement. AmaBomvane acknowledge that they are not, without the other, and this *Ubuntu* philosophy, has a strong hold in their daily life. Elders hold knowledge about caring for people with disabilities and are often seen as wisdom keepers, while community members are caretakers, not just families, providing support.

8.2.5.4 Inclusion of Persons with Disability in Xhosa Rituals

In Xhosa communities, Xhosa rituals are critical in marking the different phases of the growth of a child. It is believed that if you miss a ritual being done for you, you tend to exhibit a certain type of behaviour that is not accepted for your stage of development, e.g. bed wetting. When AmaBomvane, who consisted of persons with disabilities, and non-disabled persons were asked about the inclusion of person with disabilities in Xhosa rituals, their response was congruent with their world view. They further expanded that in KwaBomvana, the treatment of persons with disabilities is inclusive because we were all created by God and that is why they exclude no one in rituals. Persons with disabilities are like them, and not different from them, they see a person not disability.

They see that they are all equal before God and there is no special ritual for a person with a disability. When they talk about a person with a disability they are talking about a human being because the blood is the same and they are also a family member. Of importance to AmaBomvane is the spiritual component of the person. They tend to see that disability is just like a blanket any other spirit is wearing and that the soul is not disabled. The status of a person with a disability must be of no less importance and disability must not be a deterrent from performing rituals for persons with disability. They concluded by centring their argument to their traditions and their world view that allows relationships to co-exist with people with disabilities. [Contribution on inclusion of persons with disabilities in Xhosa rituals was made by: Traditional Healer, Circumcision surgeon, social worker and Parents of Persons with disabilities].

Key Points Emerging from the Case Study

- **AmaBomvane indigenous world view is encompassing and inclusive:** The tenants of AmaBomvane world view ensure that everybody including persons with disabilities are included in community life.
- **Diverse abilities are honoured by AmaBomvane:** Because of their strong bonds of being a community, what is diverse is seen as enhancing the Bomvane beingness and becoming. Not as something that must be pushed aside.

- **Rituals and ceremonies are inclusive of all community members:** Their deeper understanding of how rituals bind them as a person they ensure that all community members are included in performing rituals.
- **Ubuntu as guiding light that connects community members:** Ubuntu permeates to all sectors of society, which demands respect for all humanity, hence people with disabilities are valued and embraced.
- **AmaBomvane see disability as outside the body, a cover, not the real person:** Bomvane reminds us on what is important—the real person not the disability.

8.3 The Need to Reconceptualize Perspectives About African Disability Thinking

The above case study of AmaBomvane appears to be in contradiction from accepted views regarding disability and people of African descent. Earlier in this chapter we highlighted how lately African understanding and interpretation of disability is guided by disability thinking that have been conceptualized from Global North. As part of colonization, there was an urgent need to ensure that African thinking was cleared from the mind of the African child who needed to be educated in the imperial way of thinking and doing as Africans were seen by their colonial masters as uneducated (Mji, 2019). African Academic institutions including health science faculties, where rehabilitation practitioners are trained, were built on fundamentals of Western foundation. Sefotho (2021) argues that Indigenous ontologies have for many centuries endured epistemological subjugation from Euro-Western epistemologies. He further expands that these indigenous ontologies within the field of disability, encountered "oppressive discourses of disability" which side-lined indigenous knowledge systems.

Ohajunwa (2019) argue that disability studies, as a discipline, is driven by a knowledge system dominated by Global North narratives. The pushers of these narratives do not endeavour to consciously understand the knowledge emanating from Global South, thereby centring and universalizing Global North disability concepts. This situation has constantly negated the lived experiences of persons with disabilities in

Global South, who not only live with current challenges to inclusion, but also exist with the historical marginalization and trivialization of their lived experiences (Meekosha, 2011). This is particularly rife within African indigenous communities, where most African knowledges are marginalized.

There has been a generalized negative perception on how Africans respond to disability. African onto-epistemologies had hardly been represented in the understanding of disability and knowledge creation about it (Sefotho, 2021). Ohajunwa (2019) assets that within South African indigenous communities, the understanding of humanity, although with certain similar tenets, is positioned differently from the largely accepted definition of humanness ascribed within the human rights understanding (Ohajunwa, 2019). There is a need to understand how African indigenous communities think and conceptualize about disability and unpack the implications of these perspectives on the lived experience of these communities.

Masaka (2018) when addressing issues of colonization, calls for epistemic liberation which ought to shift from the theoretical level to consideration of how this can be practically implemented. Like AmaBomvane thinking, Grech, 2015 challenges the dominant dualistic ontology of the modern West and calls for indigenous ontology that focuses on perspectives of human relationality as an understanding of the fundamentals of life. Bezzina (2018) points to the role of indigenous knowledge in understanding and development of interventions for and with persons with disabilities. This thinking is further supported by Ned, Kpobi and Ohajunwa (2022) in their paper on thinking about mental health and spirituality from the Indigenous knowledge systems frame of reference.

African researchers and persons with disabilities need to lead the dialogue on African conceptualization on disability in Global South (Grech & Soldatic, 2016; Kolawole, 2005; Chimbala-Kalenga, 2015). Within this thinking, Mji (2019) points us to Ubuntu which has been applied within various spaces in a bid to support South Africa's young democracy, create a new collective and ethical consciousness aimed at dismantling the corrosive divisive narratives of the colonial era by governments of the past. As an indigenous ethic, Ubuntu has the capacity to support a contextually and culturally relevant reconceptualization of rights as applied to disability. This will potentially enable persons with disabilities and their families within African indigenous contexts to access rights and opportunities currently inaccessible to them. Part of reconceptualization of disability thinking in Africa is to decolonize the disability studies to align with African thinking.

8.3.1 The Use of the Backward and Forward Movement in Reconceptualization of African Disability Studies

As previously stated, there is a negative suggestion of how people of African descent view and deal with disability. Without underplaying this view, it is also important to bring to light other perspectives about how indigenous Africans view disability. The case study shared by Dwadwa-Henda (2023) and that of Sefotho's paper in 2021 highlight a need to revisit the discussion about the lens used by Africans towards disability. Contrary to the accepted norm, people of African descent appear to use inclusive norms undergirded by humanness and Ubuntu when dealing with disability. It is also important to point out the challenge of not knowing and understanding how Africans related to disability before they were colonized, except for case studies such as that of Dwadwa-Henda, (2023) and that of Sefotho, (2021). The danger of this is to start conceptualizing about African disability thinking as if one is starting from a blank slate.

In this chapter we draw from one of the indigenous scholars from kwaBomvane, Tinky-Penny in Mji (2013) who advocates for a backward and forward movement in dealing with lost indigenous knowledge systems, and whereby he advocates for indigenous scholars to use a critical lens that will question and replace what is not relevant in how Africans view disability with relevant research evidence (Mji, 2013). This then will prevent the proverbial 'throwing out the baby with the bath water'. We envisage the development of a colourful blanket that integrate and mixes both the North and West knowledge with African knowledge system.

8.4 Chapter Conclusion

The generalized perception regarding that people of African descent view disability negatively need to be reconceptualized. Other views exist that seem to challenge this view. With changes in Africa that were brought by colonization and modernity, it is difficult to know how people of African descent viewed disability before they were colonized. During this period of decolonization, there is a need to rethink and reconceptualize how people of African descent view disability. When this happens, there is a need to ensure that the baby is not thrown out with the bath water by ensuring that relevant aspects learnt from literature from Global North are kept.

References

Amanze, J.N., (2011). Contextuality: African Spirituality as a Catalyst for Spiritual Formation in Theological Education in Africa., XVI (2).

Barnes, C. (1992). Qualitative research: Valuable or irrelevant? *Disability, Handicap and Society, 7*, 139–155.

Berg, A. (2003). Ancestor Reverence and Mental Health in South Africa. In *Transcultural Psychiatry* (Vol. 40, Issue 2, pp. 194–207). https://doi.org/10.1177/1363461503402004

Bezzina, L. (2018). The role of indigenous and external knowledge in development interventions with disabled people in Burkina Faso: the implications of engaging with lived experiences. *Disability and the Global South*, *5*(2), 1488–1507. https://www.researchgate.net/publication/327012134

Bradbury-Jones, C., Ogik, P., Betts, J., Taylor, J., & Lund, P. (2018). Beliefs about people with albinism in Uganda: A qualitative study using the common-sense model. *PLoS ONE*, *13*(10). https://doi.org/10.1371/journal.pone.0205774

Bruchac, M. M. (2020). Indigenous Knowledge and Traditional Knowledge. *Encyclopedia of Global Archaeology, 5686–5696*. https://doi.org/10.1007/978-3-030-30018-0_10

Chimbala-Kalenga, R. (2015). Adjusting western research techniques to accommodate research in the indigenous realm. Indilinga: African Journal of Indigenous Knowledge Systems Vol. 14 No. 1

Chikane, F. (2012). Eight days in September: The removal of Thabo Mbeki. Johannesburg, South Africa: Picador Africa.

Chilisa, B. (2012). *Indigenous Research Methodologies*. Sage Publications Inc.

Chuengsatiansup, K. (2002). Spirituality and health: An initial proposal to incorporate spiritual health in health impact assessment. *Environmental Impact Assessment Review, 23*(1), 3–15.

Comaroff, J., & Comaroff, J. L. (2012). Theory from the south: Or, how Euro-America is evolving toward Africa. *Anthropological Forum, 22*(2), 113–131. https://doi.org/10.1080/00664677.2012.694169

Dube, A. K., & Charowa, G. (2005). Are Disabled Peoples' Voices from both South and North Being heard in the Development process? *Disabled Women Support Organisation, June.*

Dwadwa-Henda, N. (2023). *"Experiences of persons with disabilities of Xhosa rituals and traditions, which contribute to health and wellbeing", PhD thesis*

(Issue March) [Open Access, Stellenbosch University]. https://scholar.sun.ac.za/handle/10019.1/128429

Eide, A. H., Khupe, W., & Mannan, H. (2014). Development process in Africa: Poverty, politics and indigenous knowledge. *African Journal of Disability, 3*(2). https://doi.org/10.4102/ajod.v3i2.75

Ferrer, J. N. (2011). *Participatory Spirituality and Transpersonal Theory: A Ten-Year Retrospective., 43*(1), 1–34.

Grange, L. L. (2009). Are there distinctive indigenous methods of inquiry? *INDILINGA, 8*(2), 189–198.

Grech, S. (2015). Decolonising Eurocentric disability studies: Why colonialism matters in the disability and global South debate. *Social Identities, 21*(1), 6–21. https://doi.org/10.1080/13504630.2014.995347

Grech, S., & Soldatic, K. (Eds.). (2016). Disability in the Global South: The Critical Handbook. Springer International Publishing: Imprint: Springer.

Gyamfi, E. A. (2021). Defying the odds: A self-reflection of an Indigenous woman lawyer with a disability in Ghana. In *Disability Studies Quarterly* (Vol. 41, Issue 4). https://doi.org/10.18061/dsq.v41i4.8458

Inguanzo, I. (2017). *The situation of indigenous children with disabilities* (Issue January). https://www.researchgate.net/publication/322358177_The_situation_of_indigenous_children_with_disabilities

James, L.A., (2015). Indigenous Spirituality: Insights for a Life-Affirming and Life-Sustaining Economy of Life. *The Ecumenical Review*, 67(2), pp.203–207. Available at: http://doi.wiley.com/https://doi.org/10.1111/erev.12152.

Kitchin, R. (2005). *Towards Emancipatory and Empowering Disability Research: Reflections on Three Participatory Action Research Projects*. National University of Ireland Maynooth.

Kisanji, J. (1995). Interface between culture and disability in the Tanzanian context: I. *International Journal of Disability, Development and Education, 42*(2), 93–108. https://doi.org/10.1080/0156655950420202

Kolawole, D. (2005). Concepts of Politics. In D. Kolawole (Ed.), *Readings in Political Science* (pp. 1–14). Dakaal Publishers.

Leshota, P. L., & Sefotho, M. M. (2020). Being differently abled: Disability through the lens of hierarchy of binaries and Bitso-lebe-ke Seromo. *African Journal of Disability, 9*, 1–7. https://doi.org/10.4102/ajod.v9i0.643

Lubinga, E. (2014). Exploring the possibility of including African proverbs in HIV and AIDS messages to influence reception by the South African youth. *South African Journal of African Languages, 34*(supl), 15–22. https://doi.org/10.1080/02572117.2014.896527

Masaka, D. (2018). "African Philosophy and the Challenge from Hegemonic Philosophy". *Education As Change* 22 (3):22 pages. https://doi.org/10.25159/1947-9417/2918.

Masasa, T., Irwin-Carruthers, S., & Faure, M. (2005). Knowledge of, beliefs about and attitudes to disability: Implications for health professionals. *South African Family Practice, 47*(7), 40–44. https://doi.org/10.1080/20786204.2005.10873260

Meekosha, H. (2011). Decolonising disability: Thinking and acting globally. *Disability and Society, 26*(6), 667–682. https://doi.org/10.1080/09687599.2011.602860

Mji, G. (2013). *Exploring the health knowledge carried by older Xhosa women in their home situation, with special focus on Indigenous knowledge* [Stellenbosch]. https://scholar.sun.ac.za/items/4c2431c5-5387-4697-a626-8d8a781b4c3f

Mji, G. (2019). *The walk without limbs searching for Indigenous Health Knowledge in a rural context in South Africa*. AOSIS. https://library.oapen.org/handle/20.500.12657/37695

Mji, G., & Ohajunwa, C. (2021). *Ubuntu ethics and human rights: Implications for rehabilitation practices in indigenous African families of persons with disabilities (PWDs).* Midrand KR Publishing.

Ned, L (2015). Recommendations for a way forward at Stellenbosch University with regards to disability. Casual Day Report 2015 Disability Campaign.

Ned, L., Kpobi, L., & Ohajunwa, C. (2022). Thinking about mental health and spirituality from the Indigenous knowledge systems frame of reference. *Disability Studies Quarterly, 41*(4). https://doi.org/10.18061/dsq.v41i4.8450

Nyangweso, M. (2018). *Disability in Africa: A Cultural / Religious Perspective. June*. https://www.researchgate.net/publication/352486275_Disability_in_Africa_A_CulturalReligious_Perspective

Ohajunwa, C. (2019). *Understanding, interpretation and expression of spirituality and its influence on care and wellbeing: An explorative case study of a South African indigenous community. April* 1–397.

Ohajunwa, C.O. & Sefotho, M.M. (2024). Epistemologies of disability from the Global South: Towards good health. In The Routledge International Handbook of Disability and Global Health. Lieketseng Ned, Minerva Rivas Verlade, Satendra Singh, Leslie Swartz and Karen Soldatic (Eds). ISBN 9781032131849. 10,4324/9781003228059

Ohajunwa, C. O., Mji, G., & Chimbala-Kalenga, R. (2022). Encouraging reciprocal healthcare practice within a South African Indigenous community. AlterNative: An International Journal of Indigenous Peoples, 18(1), 141–146. https://doi.org/10.1177/11771801221085631

Ohajunwa, C., Mji, G., & Chimbala-Kalenga, R. (2021). Framing wellbeing through spirituality, space, history, and context: Lessons from an indigenous African community. *Wellbeing, Space and Society, 2*, Article 100042.

Oliver, M. (1992). Changing the social relations of research production. *Disability, Handicap and Society, 7*, 101–114.

Parsloe, S. M. (2015). Discourses of Disability, Narratives of Community: Reclaiming an Autistic Identity Online. *Journal of Applied Communication Research, 43*(3), 336–356. https://doi.org/10.1080/00909882.2015.1052829

Rohwerder, B. (2018). Disability stigma in developing countries. *Helpdesk Report*, 26. https://assets.publishing.service.gov.uk/media/5b18fe3240f0b634aec30791/Disability_stigma_in_developing_countries.pdf

Sefotho, M. M. (2021). Basotho ontology of disability: An afrocentric onto-epistemology. *Heliyon, 7*(3), 8. https://doi.org/10.1016/j.heliyon.2021.e06540

Smith, L. T. (2012). *Decolonizing Methodologies: Research and Indigenous Peoples*. Zed Books. https://books.google.co.za/books?id=2U0ETwEACAAJ

Stone-MacDonald, A., & Butera, G. (2012). Cultural beliefs and attitudes about disability in East Africa. *Rev of Dis Stud: An Int Journ, 8*(1), 1–19.

Talle, A. (2020). A Child Is a Child: Disability and Equality among the Kenya Maasai. In B. Ingstad & S. R. Whyte (Eds.), *Disability and Culture* (pp. 56–72). University of California Press. https://doi.org/10.1525/9780520342194-005

Tigere, B., & Moyo, T. (2022). Disability-inclusive community development: A case of a community garden in Limpopo province in South Africa. *African Journal of Disability, 11*, 1–11. https://doi.org/10.4102/AJOD.V10I0.850

United Nations. (2006). *Convention on the rights of persons with disabilities and otional protocol*. 37. https://doi.org/10.5463/DCID.v29i4.656

van Binsbergen, W. (2011). "African spirituality: An approach from intercultural philosophy" http://www.shikanda.net/african religion/spirit.htm.

Wheeler, E. A., Ampadu, L. M., & Wangari, E. (2002). Lifespan development revisited: African-centered spirituality throughout the life cycle. *Journal of Adult Development, 9*(1), 71–78.

WHO. (2001). *International Classification of Functioning*.

CHAPTER 9

The Guidance of African Thinking to Assist AfriNEAD Achieve Sustainability

Gubela Mji, *Chioma Ohajunwa*, *and Nomvo Dwadwa-Henda*

9.1 Introduction

AfriNEAD was established against the backdrop of persons with disabilities experiencing marginalization, exclusion and poverty within the African region. The aim of AfriNEAD to establish the network was to create a platform whereby a diverse "community of practice" could provide evidence and ways of using this evidence to improve the lives of persons with disabilities Africa. From the start, AfriNEAD had an ambitious agenda—it was to be an inclusive network drawing on the best skills, expertise and goodwill of researchers and disability activists. Some

G. Mji (✉) · C. Ohajunwa · N. Dwadwa-Henda
Cape Town, South Africa
e-mail: gumji@sun.ac.za

C. Ohajunwa
e-mail: chioma@sun.ac.za

N. Dwadwa-Henda
e-mail: nhenda@sun.ac.za

G. Mji (ed.), *Doing Disability Research in Africa*,
https://doi.org/10.1007/978-3-031-98549-2_9

AfriNEAD members are prominent researchers; others bring their insider knowledge of what it takes to effect changes for marginalized people in difficult contexts. While most members celebrate in this diversity, the gulf in lived experience amongst members brings its own tensions and dynamics and requires flexibility to accommodate different perspectives.

One of the key roles for leadership is to help people who may feel far from one another, to have a common sense of purpose and to value what each brings to the greater project of improving lives. This is easier said than done and is a long-term project, the outcome of which is by no means certain. The very first conference in 2007 was contentious as for the first time, persons with disabilities who have suffered severe exclusion in disability research—which is about their lives—were in the same room with disability researchers and were engaged in debates about disability research. Persons with disabilities started to challenge researchers about the pain that was caused to them by research. For example, there is the issue of eugenics (the use of selective breeding to improve humans), and though this might not mean these researchers have that type of thinking of participating in eugenics, to persons with disabilities, the whole research enterprise was a flawed entity. Persons with disabilities were deeply concerned about the lack of inclusion in disability research. On reflecting on some of the controversies, it was clear that integral to the process of developing sustainable networks within an African cosmology, was the need to pay close attention to the relationships amongst all participants, and it is in this context that this chapter we will share different pivots and turning moments on how AfriNEAD used African thinking to brave the storms and ride through to be a sustainable African disability network.

9.2 Background

The concept of networking is as old as humankind. Early on, humanity recognized the need for networking and co-opting the strengths and potential of other human beings in their day-to-day existence for survival, progress and development (Mji et al., 2009). The adage that says 'the whole is greater than the sum of its parts' also recognizes this.

Similarly, in Africa (Nguni, South Africa), we say '*Umntu ngumntu ngabantu*', (meaning: a person is a person because of other people) (Bergh, 2017). There is a general challenge of sustainability of research networks that are addressing issues about persons with disabilities. Some of these challenges are related to the fact that these networks, are externally funded by donors who do not support the networks once their funding tenure expires. Many of these externally funded research networks cannot continue without external funding. The challenge with this type of scenario in the region is the repetition of similar research questions by different donors, as donors do not conduct fact-finding about previous research that has been conducted before implementing new research programs.

This is a challenge, as the research conducted by many of the disability research projects is about the description of an aspect about disability. These types of studies exhaust persons with disabilities as it appears that they are always describing issues about themselves which is very tiring for them as they already know these issues and sometimes, it is not the first time they have been asked to describe these issues in disability research. Persons with disabilities are calling for the adoption of research strategies that are both emancipatory (seeking 'positive' societal change) and empowering (seeking 'positive' individual change through participation) (Kitchin, 2005). AfriNEAD was developed to ensure that relationships are improved between persons with disabilities and disability researchers and a door was opened for persons with disabilities to play an inclusive role that warrants them to play different roles (Mckenzie et al., 2014). The process of building up this inclusive model required AfriNEAD to be sustainable.

Persons with disabilities have been struggling for generations to achieve equity. Friedman et al. (2007) suggest that the networks aspect of social capital is also useful to best understand the active, on-the-ground processes by which people of some countries, who are beset with poverty, racial/ethnic subordination and internal divisions (arising from inequalities at different levels), defend their own and others' rights and human dignity. AfriNEAD wanted to bring groups from different constituencies and network how working together as one group could hasten the realization of rights of persons with disabilities in the region.

For AfriNEAD there was a hope that coming together will scale up the effectiveness of the existing resources and achieve equitable distribution of limited resources (Daar et al., 2007; De Bont et al., 2007; Lau, 2004; Mozunder & Marathe, 2007). It has been shown by McCarthy et al. (2008) that one can possibly reach close to three million cancer patients through cancer management network teams for the dissemination of information related to palliative management. AfriNEAD has noticed that there is a challenge of distribution of disability research which ends up being stored without use in the cupboards of researchers. However, the goal of AfriNEAD was to facilitate that this research ultimately reaches the hands of people that can make a change in the lives of persons with disabilities.

Within these discussions and innovative strategies, scholars such as Duma, Tshabalala and Mji (2021) are calling for the inclusion of the voices of mothers of children with disabilities. They come with a wealth of knowledge and innovative networkers with reservoirs of prior knowledge in activities that require non-linear patterns (such as social capital) and coming together with a common purpose for problem-solving. These are some of the assets they have used in day-to-day challenges of raising children with disabilities (Duma et al., 2021).

Networks also run the risk by some members conducting parallel activities that are like the intention of the network at different levels which do not give feedback to the network, which might result in weakening the network (Mji et al., 2009). The most effective interventions by network members are those that harmonize with visions and strategies of the system of reference, in this case the network. The aim is not the realization of individual activities but strategic feedback on relationships in all measures that is supposed to create equality in the directedness of all activities. In attempting to understand how networks can achieve sustainability, we draw information from Kaplan's (1999) paper on organizational capacity.

9.2.1 Kaplan's Framework for Organizational Capacity

According to Kaplan (1999) each organization is an entity, but not entirely; it interacts with its environment, it affects and is affected by that environment. It is one entity amongst many, and its specific identity is a combination of its own internal integrity and its relationship with others. The continued growth, and the life of the organization, depends largely on its interaction with its ever-changing context and environment. Without such interaction the organization, like a biological organism—would soon become dormant and cease to function. According to Kaplan (1999) on elements of organizational capacity, six elements are presented that help organizations to achieve sustainability, and these elements are presented in Fig. 10.1 (Fig. 9.1).

Kaplan's framework for organizational capacity is explained as follows:

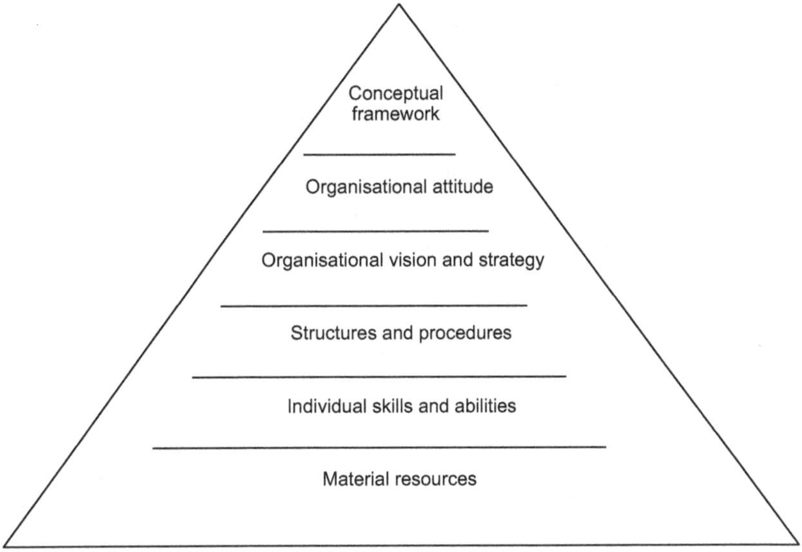
Conceptual
framework
Organisational attitude
Organisational vision and strategy
Structures and procedures
Individual skills and abilities
Material resources

Fig. 9.1 Elements of organizational capacity

A. **The** ***conceptual framework*** reflects the organization's understanding of the world. This is a coherent frame of reference, a set of concepts which allows the organization to make sense of the world around it, to locate itself within that world, and to make decisions in relation to it. This framework is not a particular ideology or theory, it is not necessarily correct, and it is not impervious to critique and change.

B. ***The organizational attitude*** incorporates the confidence to act in and on the world in a way that the organization believes to be effective and to have an impact, while accepting responsibility for social and physical conditions 'out there'. An organization needs to build its confidence to act in and on the world in a way that it believes can be effective and have an impact. Put another way, it must shift from 'playing the victim' to exerting some control, to believing in its own capacity to affect its circumstances. Another aspect of 'attitude' is accepting responsibility for the social and physical conditions 'out there', despite whatever the organization faces in the world. This implies a shift from a demand or blame-focused mentality to a more inclusive acceptance of the responsibilities which go with the recognition of human rights.

C. **The *organizational vision and strategy*** provide a sense of purpose and flows out of the understanding and responsibility of the organizational attitude. Understanding and responsibility lead to a sense of purpose in which the organization does not lurch from one problem to the next but manages to plan and implement a programme of action and is able to adapt the programme in a rational and considered manner. Organizational vision is developed, really, through an interplay between internal and external constraints and possibilities. There is a reality out there which must be responded to, and there is an inner inspiration which must be harnessed and focused.
D. ***Organizational structures and procedures*** are defined and differentiated to reflect and support vision and strategy.
E. ***Individual skills, abilities and competencies*** are relevant to the task at hand.
F. ***Material resources*** should be sufficient and appropriate.

According to Kaplan, the first three items in the triangle, i.e. the conceptual framework, the organizational attitude and vision and strategy are critical for organizations capacity and for sustainability to occur. He maintains that the last three items automatically follow once the first three are operationalized and are running smoothly.

In short, the elements at the top of the hierarchy of elements of organizational life are ephemeral, transitory, not easily assessed or weighed. They are largely invisible: invisible both to the organization itself as well as to those managers and practitioners who would intervene to build organizational capacity. Thus, the most important elements in organizational life, those which largely determine the functioning of an organization, are the elements which lie at the top of the hierarchy, not those which lie at the bottom. It is the less tangible, more invisible aspects of organizational life which largely determine organizational functioning and sustainable.

Within AfriNEAD the overarching understanding was that persons with disabilities within the African the region are struggling from marginalization. The vision of AfriNEAD is that it will be an inclusive network that brings together people of different views to focus on how the network will use research evidence as a prong for the realizations of rights of persons with disabilities. The goal is to impact policies that will cause change in the lives of persons with disabilities. Persons with disabilities are sceptical about the whole research enterprise due to experience on how research was in the past used. There exists a deep mistrust between persons with disabilities and disability researchers. To address Kaplan's (1999) top three areas of organizational capacity, organically the network started using some strategies in which, when one reflects, it became clear that some were drawn from the African way of thinking and philosophies. It became clear to the AfriNEAD Secretariat and Chairperson that over and above the challenges of building the network by ensuring that administrative functions run smoothly, an African thinking and approach might be necessary to bring stability and assist the network to focus on common purpose. The next session will present some information on the African thinking, this will be followed by the influence of some African thinking to AfriNEAD, and the chapter finishes with a chapter conclusion.

9.3 African Way of Thinking

African way of thinking is grounded in simply the way Africans perceive, conceive and contemplate their universe; the lens through which they see reality, which affects their value systems (Karangi, 2019). Although the continent of Africa has been vastly influenced by the North and the West, she continues to draw most of her values from an indigenous thinking. This approach helps one to understand the present situation by revisiting the past. In so doing, one can understand the past, the present and predict the future (Kanu, 2013). What undergirds African thinking is relationships and familyhood, reciprocity, respect and compensatory and restorative justice (Mbiti, 1969). Undergirding this approach is the concept of Ubuntu. There is a perception that Africans never forget their thinking even if they are removed from their origins and that this thinking just gets pushed into the unconscious: critical incidences such as illnesses make them revert to that original thinking (Maelene, 2002).

African thinking and philosophies are a broad subject, and it would be a challenge to try and cover them all in this chapter. AfriNEAD mainly used Ubuntu as an umbrella that undergirded African thinking in assisting AfriNEAD to achieve some of the intangible aspects of organizational culture and be sustainability. To keep the network focused on its intention of being a sustainable network, there was a need to ensure that Kaplan's top three areas of organizational capacity were operationalized, and Ubuntu seemed to be an appropriate umbrella in supporting the network. Though Ubuntu has been described in the previous chapter, in this chapter we intend to revisit the discussion on Ubuntu and highlight some key tenets of this African philosophy as follows.

9.3.1 Key Tenets of Ubuntu

Ubuntu values humanity, without it, people lose being humans and become animals (Kaunda, 1966; Ramose, 2003; Wiredu, 1980). Ubuntu challenges the concept that you can become human, while those around you are not regarded as humans (Umuntu ngumuntu ngabantu). For a person to become human, one considers others and allows oneself to become one with others and become a person/people and to develop relationships that create strong communal boards (Mbiti, 1969). When one allows the self to become one with others, this might imply letting go of the external coat, as Dwadwa-Henda (2023) study amongst Bomvane people has shown, that the most important aspect is not the body but the soul.

One of the important attributes of Ubuntu is the acknowledgement of everybody, thereby by including everybody, by making visible the invisible, and this is at the core of addressing the deep concern of persons with disabilities who have been ignored by society. In many ways, an understanding of Ubuntu, is about moving away from artificial differences between people and creating an enabling environment of dignity (Bergh, 2017). The collectivists and communality assist in developing united families with healthy relationships. This shared collective humanness or social ethics is what has assisted Africans during colonialism and apartheid in South Africa (Bergh, 2017) and this chimes closely to what was required by AfriNEAD to create a united network. People of African descent see unity as strength and frown upon individual approaches that creates the "them" and "us".

Persons with disabilities in their grassroots struggle against oppression and disablement in the twentieth century have been fighting for their humanity, when disability was still viewed as a demarcated issue and not a part of enabling a human diversity, as argued in African understandings of Ubuntu (Bergh, 2017). Dwadwa-Henda (2023) explains how AmaBomvane, an indigenous community in the Eastern Cape Province of South Africa, negate the binaries of describing some of their family members as disabled and abled as, according to them, from time-to-time some family members do struggle from some form of functionality problems, and this does not mean a special name of disability must now be assigned to them.

The cultural principle of Ubuntu (as used in South Africa, or other linguistic variations used throughout Africa) refers to a social system of interrelatedness whereby people's humanity is determined not by their personal qualities, but in terms of how they relate to all in their community (Bergh, 2017; Boon, 1996). The idea that 'a person is a person through other persons' encapsulates the essence of the Ubuntu philosophy, contrasting sharply with more individualized Western views. In this regard the notion that persons with disabilities should strive for 'independence' is called into question and the questioning of this notion is further supported by Mji and Ohajunwa (2021) in their chapter on Ubuntu ethics and human rights: Implications for rehabilitation practices in indigenous African families of persons with disabilities. Ubuntu is a more interconnected way of being which locates people not as independent individuals striving for self-actualization, but as interdependent beings who are part of a collective, who derive their sense of identity and recognition by contributing to the development of others and improving the common good of "all" (Mbigi & Maree, 1995). AfriNEAD adopted Ubuntu as a guiding tool for its day-to-day operations and to answer challenges and contesting issues that faced the network from a point of compassion. This decision above aligns with the dual aspects of Ubuntu, as a philosophy, and a practical strategy of human engagement.

Below are key tenets of Ubuntu that were used to support AfriNEAD to become a sustainable network:

9.3.1.1 Key Tenets of Ubuntu That Influenced the Sustainability of AfriNEAD

This section presents key tenets of Ubuntu that influence sustainability of AfriNEAD, and these are: Relationships as a glue for sustainability, this is followed by the collective as opposed to individualism, Ubuntu and disability as changing social constructs is outlined, the final aspect of the section is Development of a disability research community of practice.

Relationships as a Glue for Sustainability

Samuel et al. (2014) proposed that relationships from an African perspective are defined in interconnectedness, interdependence, sense of solidarity and belongingness. Social connectedness lies at the heart of care and support of African people (Stavrova & Luhmann, 2016). Thus, the relational nature of African cultures includes "wholeness, community, and harmony, which are deeply embedded in cultural values" (Owusu-Ansah & Mji, 2013, p. 2). Relationships and interconnectedness play an important role in African worldviews (Owusu-Ansah & Mji, 2013; Helne & Hirvilammi, 2015). Owusu-Ansah and Mji (2013) further contend that a person pursues individual and collective harmony to become a whole person.

Given that AfriNEAD's vision was to develop a united network that brings together diverse groups of people, it was possible to foresee two potential threats to the process of developing a sustainable network. There was a danger in focusing on the last three elements of Kaplan's (1999) framework which would be for AfriNEAD to focus on, an entirely technicist and outputs-based approach to research which could undermine those intangible aspects and threaten the sense of common purpose and diverse contributions that currently exist within AfriNEAD. There was also fear from hard core researchers that AfriNEAD might focus too much on process and commonalities which could create a self-referential group that misses the opportunity to take on the difficult challenges of providing good data to move evidence into action.

It was clear that AfriNEAD would have to opt for the intangibles in the hope of keeping the group together and for persons with disabilities to develop trust. This was in order that persons with disabilities would open and share their life stories and experiences of being disabled. With this, the hope that it would assist in strengthening a community-centred and African approach to what is often seen as an individualistic, technical and competitive challenge which may create opportunities for all to learn from one another and as a group, develop the network.

The Collective as Opposed to Individualism

In the African indigenous world, no one is 'independent', and no human being is alone. This is why Africans do not promote the cartesian cogito ergo sum (I think therefore I am) but the existential cognatus sum, ergo sums (I am known therefore we are). This is well manifested through various rituals especially those of naming, important rites of passage, as well as genuine communion with the ancestors (Dwadwa-Henda, 2023). This approach assists in building communities of trust which enhance unity and the ability for communities to see themselves as the collective. This trust enhances resilience and helps in building up communities of life. In contrast, to see challenges in trying to unify opposing ideas, AfriNEAD accepted diversity and social inclusiveness as part of a growing network (Mji et al., 2011). There was a general caution about Western concepts of disability that emphasize medical issues and that with their divisive approach may be inadequate to achieve the inclusiveness AfriNEAD was focusing on (Mji et al., 2011).

As earlier stated, the cultural principle of Ubuntu (as used in South Africa, or other linguistic variations used throughout Africa) refers to a social system of interrelatedness whereby people's humanity is determined not by their personal qualities, but in terms of how they relate to all in their community (Boon, 1996). The idea that 'a person is a person through other persons' encapsulates the essence of the Ubuntu philosophy, contrasting sharply with more individualized western views. In this regard the notion that persons with disabilities should strive for 'independence' is called into question. Ubuntu is a more interconnected way of being which locates people not as independent individuals striving for self-actualization, but as interdependent beings who are part of a collective, who derive their sense of identity and recognition by contributing to the development of others and improving the common good of 'all' (Mbigi & Maree, 1995).

More importantly, total inclusion of indigenous persons with disabilities in research based on mutual respect, such as suggested by the Afrocentric method, solidifies participants' own definition of self-determination and empowerment. Fostering self-esteem and empowerment are particularly important in disability research because of the close link between disability and poverty (Mji et al., 2011). Disability, made worse by poverty, robs people of their dignity and sense of self. In a situation such as this, research that simply treats participants as 'outsiders' can only fuel an already eroded and fragile sense of self. The AfriNEAD organizational attitude is to see its membership as a collective with each having something to contribute to the sustainability of the network.

Lastly, there is a need within AfriNEAD to ensure that the voices of African persons with disabilities led the discussions in building up an African understanding of disability as they had the lived experiences of being disabled. As mentioned in the previous chapter, there is a paucity in literature regarding how Africans conceptualize disability. Existing literature paints a negative picture of how people of African descent respond to disability. These discussions would contribute to the development and conceptualization of African theories which can start influencing disability programs in African universities that run disability studies. Within Africa, there is a multiplicity of understandings given to disability, based on both the diverse contexts and belief systems, as well as the varied experiences that various African indigenous communities have been subjected to (Mji & Ohajunwa, 2021). In terms of oral history, medical and missionary, mainly Western, influences of segregation and categorization, and definitions ascribed by various world international instruments and funding organizations still impact these communities. These categorizations neglect the more collectivist approaches favoured within these indigenous communities.

Development of a Disability Research 'Community of Practice'

In African communities, a community is emphasized more than a member's individuality, and this creates a chain of interrelationships. The first item that warranted AfriNEAD sustainability is the diverse "community of practice" that AfriNEAD congregated to provide evidence and ways of using this evidence to improve the lives of persons with disabilities in Africa. AfriNEAD has an ambitious agenda of wanting to be an inclusive network drawing on the best skills and expertise as well as the goodwill of everyone who can contribute something on disability research. While it is good to have this diversity, the gulf of lived experiences between AfriNEAD stakeholders initially created contesting debates that required time for the stakeholders to realize that their views regarding how to solve the challenges facing persons with disabilities might be different, all were aiming for the same goal. They needed to develop a united front to challenge the systems that have contributed to the marginalization of persons with disabilities within the region. This building of communities of trust within AfriNEAD required time to consolidate.

AfriNEAD noticed that even four years after its inauguration, there were still elements of mistrust amongst its membership. Therefore, AfriNEAD opted to specifically dialogue on the issue of trust amongst its membership by first ensuring that the 2011 conference was entitled: Building Communities of Trust. AfriNEAD followed this by assigning one of the respected stakeholders who was a person with disability late Dr Rachel Kachaje to deliver a keynote address on this topic. Alternating roles and encouraging persons with disabilities to play leading roles in research and sometimes taking over mediating roles on how disability could be further supported in academic institutions by persons with disabilities. This started to create confidence that academic researchers could hand over some critical responsibilities to be managed by persons with disabilities.

Ubuntu and Disability as Changing Social Constructs

Ubuntu has become an instrument used in examining the social and cultural history of the African continent which tells a completely different story and illustrates how Africans have formulated and shaped theories as well as actions of decolonization and relationships to disability in their own epistemological and transnational terms (Bergh, 2017).

Ubuntu is an African humanist and ethical world view, and within which exists disability, as part of a common humanity which is necessarily part of what makes us human. Ubuntu regarding its utility can alter over time with changes in the environment as Ubuntu recognizes difference of experiences of diversity of humanness (as positive or negative), which are part of our shared humanity (Bergh, 2017). Ubuntu is always ready to respond, change and align itself to this fluidity of human nature.

Within the network there was a general realization that persons with disabilities from Africa are products of social constructs which influences and deeply affect their lives and gives them their indigenous roots and value systems (Maathai, 2009; Mji et al., 2009). Some of these indigenous roots and value systems might include aspects such as *ubude abuphangwa* (you cannot hurry to be tall—in other words do not try to be what you have not achieved) and *uhambo alunqgitywa ngemini enye* (you do not finish a journey in one day—in other words be patient—do not try to achieve it all in one go as you might miss some learning lessons on the way as you are hurrying it all up). In the early days of the development of the network we were aware that years of oppression of persons with disabilities will not be changed overnight by the development of the network: it is these core principles that assisted the network to continue, even during challenging times, and to subdue some impatient network members who needed quick fixes (Maathai, 2009; Maelene, 2002; Mkhize, 1973).

As network members we were aware of past, including tenacious relationships between persons with disabilities and disability researchers. However contrary to Maelene (2002), our intention was not to gravitate on past relationships. As a network we were careful of solving critical incidences using fighting approaches that have been developed in the past as a response to stress created by the medical model which was creating divisions between disability researchers and persons with disabilities (Maathai, 2009; Maelene, 2002; Mkhize, 1973). These divisions were about the "them" and "us" and at the core of these approaches was a response to scarce resources. These methods are of struggle for self-preservation and protecting one's territory: they do not define us as African peoples and create a buffer between us and Ubuntu (Chikane, 2012; Mbeki, 1996; Mji, 2012). We knew that, as a network, once we started defining ourselves with such value systems, we would lose our human value systems (*umntu ngumuntu ngabantu*) (Some, 1994; Berghs, 2017; Boon, 1996) and become vulnerable and broken without achieving our vision of being a sustainable network. If we were to build an inclusive network that puts our actions for those that are struggling first when solving challenges (SA INDS, 1997), such approaches for self- preservation and protecting one's territory will not have a place in AfriNEAD. Instead—as a network—we will continue to draw strength and resilience using concepts such as Ubuntu.

Key Aspects That Emerged on This Section
Kaplan (1995) highlighted the need to focus on intangible aspects for an organization to be sustainable. AfriNEAD acknowledges the differences of the past between persons with disabilities and disability researchers. These differences, if ignored, could create more divisions within the network. Drawing from the African thinking, AfriNEAD used Ubuntu tenets to assist the network to become sustainable.

9.4 Chapter Conclusion

AfriNEAD is aware of varying views on disability research issues and the differing capabilities in the field of disability research. AfriNEAD chose Ubuntu as an organizing principle to guide respectful engagement amongst people with widely differing skills and experiences with the overall project of collaborating in research and development to make a positive difference to persons with disabilities. Using Kaplan (1999) framework of organizational capacity to guide the network on elements of building capacity for sustainable organizations, AfriNEAD chose Ubuntu as a vehicle to bind differences and to unite the network. African thinking could be a resource that could assist in creating resilient disability networks. This thinking could further be a springboard and provide guidance in the African understanding of disability.

References

Bergh, M. (2017). Practices and discourses of Ubuntu: Implications for an African model of disability? *African Journal of Disability, 6*, 292.

Boon, M. (1996). *The African way. The power of interactive leadership*. Struik Publishers.

Chikane, F. (2012). Eight days in September: The removal of Thabo Mbeki. Johannesburg, South Africa: Picador Africa.

Daar, A. S., Berndtson, K., Persad, D. L., & Singer, P. A. (2007, 3 December). How can developing countries harness biotechnology to improve health? *BMC Public Health, 7,* 346.

De Bont, A., Stoevelaar, H., & Bal, R. (2007, 7 December). Databases as policy instruments. About extending networks as evidence-based policy. *MBC Health Serv. Res., 7*, 200.

Dwadwa-Henda, N. (2023). *"Experiences of persons with disabilities of Xhosa rituals and traditions, which contribute to health and wellbeing", PhD thesis* (Issue March) [Open Access, Stellenbosch University]. https://scholar.sun.ac.za/handle/10019.1/128429

Duma, V., Tshabalala, N., & Mji, G. (2021). The black hole of dealing with a disability diagnosis: Views of South African rural parents Afr. *J Disability, 10,* 951. Published online 2021 Nov 29. https://doi.org/10.4102/AJOD.v10i0.951

Friedman, S. R., Mateu-Gelabert, P., Curtis, R., Maslow, C., Bolyard, M., Sandoval, M., & Flom, P. L. (2007, June). Social capital or networks, negotiations, and norms? Neighbourhood case study. *Am J Prev. Med., 32* (6 Supplement), S160–70.

Helne, T., & Hirvilammi, T. (2015). Wellbeing and sustainability: A relational approach. *Sustainable Development, 23*(3), 167–175. https://doi.org/10.1002/sd.1581

Kanu, I. A. (2013). On the sources of African philosophy. *Filosofia Theoretica: Journal of African Philosophy, Culture and Religions, 2*(1), 337–402.

Karangi, M. M. (2019). African cosmology. *Research Gate*. https://doi.org/10.13140/RG.2.2.35377.74082

Kaplan, A. (1999). *The development of capacity.* UN non-governmental liaison service (NGLS): Switzerland and New York.

Kaunda, K. D. (1966) *A Humanist in Africa* by London, Longmans Green, pp. 136. I5s.

Kitchin, R. (2005). *Towards emancipatory and empowering disability research: Reflections on three participatory action research projects*. National University of Ireland Maynooth.

Lau, F. (2004, 20 September). Towards a conceptual knowledge management framework in health. *Perspect Health Inf manag., 1*, 8.

Maathai, W. (2009). *The challenge for Africa: A new vision*. The Random House Group Limited.

Maelene, M. (2002). Implications of indigenous African beliefs and customs for health education and prevention of HIV/AIDS. *Nutrition Update, 26*(8), 14–17.

Mbeki, G. (1996). *Sunset at midday*. Nolwazi Educational Publishers.

Mbigi, L., & Maree, J. (1995). *Ubuntu. The spirit of African transformation management*. Knowledge Resources.

Mbiti, J. (1969). *African religions and philosophy*. Anchor Books.

McCarthy, M., Gonzalez- Izquierdo, A., Sherlaw- Jonson, C., & Khachatryn, A. (2008). A comparative indicator for cancer networks in England: Availability, characteristics and presentation. *BMC Health Services research. 8*(1):45

McKenzie, J., Mji, G., & Gcaza, S. (2014). With or without us? An audit of disability research in the southern African region. *AJOD, 3* (2).

Mji, G., Gcaza, S., Melling–Williams, N., & MacLachlan, M. (2009). Networking in disability for development: Introducing the African Network For Evidence-to-action on disability. In M. MacLachlan & L. Swartz (Eds.),*Disability, and international development towards inclusive global health*. Springer, pp. 69–89.

Mji, G., Gcaza, S., Swartz, L., MacLachlan, M., & Hutton, B. (2011). An African way of networking around disability. *Disability and Society; 26*(3).

Mji, G. (2012). *The health knowledge utilised by rural older Xhosa women in the management of health problems in their home situation, with a special focus on indigenous knowledge [Doctoral Thesis]*. University of Stellenbosch.

Mji, G., & Ohajunwa, C. (2021). *Ubuntu ethics and human rights: Implications for rehabilitation practices in indigenous African families of persons with disabilities (PWDs)*. Midrand KR Publishing.

Mkhize, N. (1973). Psychology: An African perspective. In: D. Hook (Ed.), *Critical psychology*. UCT Press.

Mozunder, P., & Marathe, A. (2007, 10 October). Role of information networks in malaria survival. *Malaria Journal, 6*, 136.

Ohajunwa, C. (2019). *Understanding, interpretation and expression of spirituality and its influence on care and wellbeing: An explorative case study of a South African indigenous community. April* 1–397.

Owusu-Ansah, F. E., & Mji, G. (2013). African indigenous knowledge and research. *African Journal of Disability, 2*(1), 30–35. https://doi.org/10.4102/AJOD.v2i1.30

Ramose, M. (2003). The ethics of Ubuntu. In P. Coetzee & A. Roux (Eds.), *The African philosophy reader* (pp. 324–333). Routledge.

Samuel, A. A., Reddy, B. S., & Nair, J. (2014). Conceptualizing dimensions of enterprise resource planning systems success: A socio technical perspective. *International Journal of Enterprise Information Systems, 10*, 53–75.

South African Integrated National Disability Strategy White Paper. (1997). Retrieved 7 August, 2023, from http://www.info.gov.za/whitepapers/1997/disability.htm

Stavrova, O., & Luhmann, M. (2016). Social connectedness as a source and consequence of meaning in life. *The Journal of Positive Psychology, 11*(5), 470–479. https://doi.org/10.1080/17439760.2015.1117127

View, M. N. (2011). Domestic violence research: Expanding understandings but limited perspective. *Feminist Review*. https://doi.org/10.1057/fr.2011.27

Wiredu, K. (1980). *Philosophy and an African culture: The Case of the Akan*. Cambridge University Press.

CHAPTER 10

The Future of Disability Research in Africa

Gubela Mji

10.1 Introduction

Disability is changing dramatically from a charitable, paternalistic and biomedical-based 'caring-for' persons with disability approach, to one that recognizes the human rights of persons disabilities, and their need for advocacy and empowerment, to realize the goal of genuine participation and inclusion in society. The main drivers of this change have been persons with disabilities who contributed to each milestone that has improved situations for persons with disabilities (Kachaje et al., 2014; Phiri, 2014).

The inclusion of marginalized and disadvantaged groups is a touchstone of many country constitutions globally. These constitutions have started influencing countries to have policies that could better the lives of persons with disabilities. The challenge is how to ensure that these policies are translated to action that will improve the lives of persons with disabilities. The development of a network that addresses the challenges of turning research evidence into meaningful action in disability, on an Africa-wide basis, is a particularly valuable opportunity for the region, to

G. Mji (✉)
Cape Town, South Africa
e-mail: gumji@sun.ac.za

G. Mji (ed.), *Doing Disability Research in Africa*,
https://doi.org/10.1007/978-3-031-98549-2_10

provide leadership in this area (Mji & Edusei, 2019; Mji et al., 2009). The earlier chapters in this book have painted a tapestry of a network with a conscious mind set by paying particular attention to issues of human rights and dignity.

It is difficult to speak of Africans without touching on the issue of colonization and its negative impact on African peoples including those with disability. Available literature tends to paint a negative picture on how people of African descent respond to disability. Some African scholars are calling for these suggestions to be questioned (Dwadwa-Hendȧ, 2023; Sefotho, 2021). Grech (2015) shares concerns on the fact that most persons with disabilities are in the Global South with the bulk in rural areas where they suffer the brunt of disproportionate poverty. She challenges the notion that disability studies remains profoundly influenced by West European and North American theories which focused exclusively on urban post-industrialist settings. The focus of these theories and tenets are on the social model of disability and are consistently exported to Global South that never aims to address this. This raises questions whether such models could assist in the development of policies for persons with disabilities in the Global South and breakdown existing stalemate that is about equity for persons with disabilities within the region.

When we speak of emancipation of disability research in AfriNEAD from whom must this disability research be emancipated and decolonized from? Ned et al. (2022) point to critical perspectives that requires recognition of multilayered dynamics of epistemic and political power, between individuals with and without disabilities, resourced and under-resourced contexts, and between other intersecting axes of privilege and oppression operating in specific localities, concerning race, ethnicity and gender, amongst others. Ned et al. (2022) call for sustained reflection that will help to avoid the reproduction and reinforcement of exclusionary practices that confront persons with disabilities in Africa.

The aim of this chapter is to create a way forward for the future of disability research in Africa. The intention is to use guidance from the AfriNEAD conferences resolutions (2009–2023) on research evidence and utilization; the contribution of collective ideas from research resolutions of the five conferences was seen as the best way to forge a way forward for the future of disability research in the region.

The next section of the chapter will give background, this will be followed by key themes that emerged from the AfriNEAD conferences

(2009–2023), followed by discussion and the chapter ends with a chapter conclusion.

10.2 Background

Swartz (2014) acknowledges the enormous strides in disability research from the Global South over the past few years, and there is every sign that disability research is alive, well and growing in this part of the world. He supports his argument with examples of various initiatives that are focusing on disability research. He concludes by posing a central question on how do disability researchers in our region retain the distinctive strengths which come from working in our contexts, while at the same time developing the quality and depth required in disability research that could contribute to change in people's lives for the better?

The late Mr Phiri (2014) asserts that we need to recognize that the area of disability research always raises some important and perhaps uncomfortable questions about who is and who should be driving the research agenda in Africa? In driving the research process in Africa, we have high-income and low-income countries who play different roles in disability research. This raises other concerns about the relevancy of research approaches and methodologies. Moreover, Ned et al. (2022) advocates for inclusion of persons with disabilities, not only as a civil rights issue but also to enhance the scientific integrity and interpretability of research findings to the realm of policy applications through use of accessible research design.

Indigenous scholars from Madwaleni in Elliot dale in the Eastern Cape Province of South Africa, frown upon research aims and questions that have excluded research participants in their development. To them this seems to suggest that researchers enter the research areas with already formed answers (Dwadwa-Henda, 2023). There is also the issue of relationship between persons with disabilities and the abled bodied researchers. A cohort of disabled researchers are emerging to take their rightful position in disability research. What type of relationships will develop between disability researchers and those without disability? AfriNEAD advocated for inclusive relationships that are undergird by Ubuntu (Mji & Edusei, 2019; Mji & Ohajunwa, 2022; Botha & Ohajunwa, 2024). This is further supported by late Dr Rachel Kachaje who encourages partnerships in disability research to accelerate development of conducive relationships between persons with disabilities and disability researchers (Kachaje et al., 2014). Botha and Ohajunwa (2024) are advocating for a decolonisation of the mind and the research processes, where collaborators and partners from the Global North are often more sought after than Africa-wide collaborators and this need to be addressed. Ohajunwa and Sefotho (2024) are calling for the conceptualization of disability in Africa drawing from the context. There is a call for disability epistemologies to be guided by and led by indigenous philosophies that already exist in Africa (Masaka, 2018; Ohajunwa & Sefotho, 2024). These are some of the debates about disability research in the region.

To conclude this section, Ohajunwa et al. (2022) posit that disability research and disability studies, are complicated dynamics of power and privilege and compounded by the fact that disability is a cross-cutting experience. It is necessary, therefore, to pay careful attention to the politics of voice within disability studies, the foregrounding of disability standpoint perspectives, the capacitation of scholars with disability and the dismantling of disabling barriers within that prevent persons with disabilities to achieve their full potential. The next section presents lessons learnt for the future of disability research drawn from the AfriNEAD conference resolutions.

10.3 Lessons Learnt for the Future of Disability Research from AfriNEAD Conference Resolutions

The AfriNEAD resolutions on research evidence and utilization were seen as the best way for this book to forge a way forward for the future of disability research in the region. The conference resolutions of the five conferences from 2009 to 2023 were visited to draw emerging themes. The conference that was left out was that of 2007 because at that time AfriNEAD has not started using the thematic areas drawn from the UNCRPD and that of 2020 as conference participants requested the commission on research evidence and utilization to be presented in plenary. From the five conferences, there were 49 papers presented on research evidence and utilization. The resolutions are critical research outcomes from research papers presented in the conferences and are presented in plenary after the people have presented their papers. Suggesting a way forward for the future of disability research in the African region using these resolutions seem to be appropriate as these suggestions are coming from the collective instead of one person. Below are the key themes that emerged from the resolutions.

10.3.1 *The Value of Using Different Methods in Disability Research*

Participants from these commissions felt that disability research should include qualitative, quantitative and mixed methods to produce data that could fully address the problems experienced by persons with disabilities. They felt that there is limited quantitative data on disability issues as many studies are qualitative in nature. Qualitative methods with small sample size and in-depth exploration and description to empower persons with disabilities and provide explanations which helps in the building on African disability theories, while quantitative methods assist in providing the much-needed statistics. There is a need to do proper research planning and to choose the most appropriate research methods for findings to be robust, e.g. randomized control trials (RCTs), systematic reviews, etc. When necessary large-scale studies (such as surveys) that provide information on the extent of the issues and problems are important in influencing policy changes where there is a need for numbers to illuminate the gravity and extent of the problem. There is the need to recognize and value alternative forms of gathering information to complement rigorous scientific methodologies.

10.3.2 *Participatory Emancipatory Research Methodology*

There is a cohort of disability researchers who seem to prefer participatory emancipatory methodologies. This type of research method assists one to understand the ground level experiences and contextually relevant information of participants. There is an option of bringing to the table all types of persons with or without disabilities. Researchers noted that collaboration and partnerships in research were mainly happening between international and African partners. There should be more collaborative research across all African regions. When Disabled People's Organizations (DPOs) are equal partners in research and service provision, we would provide capacity building and inclusive programmes to ensure that they do not feel left behind. When conducting reviews of disability research to understand the evidence in a local area, it is encouraged to use locally based groups to review and engage with literature about disability, disability-related topics, rehabilitation services and other topics of concern for that area as they carry authentic understanding of the data regarding their area. Researchers and local communities can jointly develop research, and this process equalizes power and practical thinking about implementation of research. There are also challenges with participatory research and some of these challenges are related to lengthy periods of negotiations with the community as it is not wise to assume that the community either always wants involvement or control (or never wants involvement or control). Within participatory research, other disability researchers and practitioners were proposing guidelines for compensation and reimbursement of research participants with disabilities. Others reported how such guidelines were developed alongside persons with disabilities, to promote the research participation of persons with disabilities and to counter the exclusion and silencing of disability voices in research. These researchers and practitioners concluded that consideration of the outlined processes in the guidelines will contribute to effectiveness and fairness of compensation and reimbursement.

10.3.3 Decolonizing Disability Research

Researchers from the region are calling for decolonization of disability research. They were committed to undertake research plans based on their own African theories, understanding and promotion of indigenous knowledge systems as a source of information. They recognized and affirmed the African homes and rural areas as creators and reservoirs of African knowledge. Using critical discursive inquiry, this assist persons with disabilities in attaining their rightful citizen position. Research and documentation should focus on African perspectives on disability (African models) that promotes indigenous knowledge systems.

The decolonization of research from the Global South through facilitating the participation and re) centring other voices and narratives of belonging could be useful in expression of voices from the children in novel and creative ways as co-researchers. This could include research methods such as poetic inquiry, arts-based inquiry and digital storytelling. Other decolonizing methodologies include creative thinking and reflection. The challenge with these methods is that they are time consuming. Once research is put into action—there need to be ongoing monitoring and evaluation to ensure that practice remains linked to evidence and appropriate to culture setting for continued effective outcomes.

Lastly disability researchers and practitioners advocated for disability research to be aligned with Ubuntu. Governments that have ratified the U.N. Convention on the Rights of Persons with Disabilities (UNCRPD) need to plan programs that relate to all the articles of the convention, guided by the human rights approach and *Ubuntu*, and particularly to respond to evidence that highlights the need for education, health, accessibility, employment creation and international cooperation. They requested that the African Union (AU) (and all its organs), Regional Economic Commissions and legislative structures should, based on *Ubuntu* principles, implement all AU Charters and Protocols that have a bearing on the lives of persons with disabilities, including the proclamation/strategies for the African Decade of Persons with Disabilities—Ubuntu should underpin all these entities.

10.3.4 Research Skills Development

There was a perception from disability researchers and practitioners that the key ingredient in advancing the inclusion of persons with disabilities was skills development and programs that strengthen self-esteem and confidence, be self-critical and to recognize the limits of what one does. The confidence to listen, read, learn a range of skills, experience and abilities that are available amongst colleagues. There was a perception that there is a need for wider dissemination of research skills within AfriNEAD. Some of these skills are about reading and understanding research literature. While supporting persons with disabilities with research skills, it is also important for researchers to understand language that has been used to address persons with disabilities in different contexts as language is a key issue underlying much of the experiences of persons with disabilities feelings of exclusion and this comes in a range of derogatory terms with regard to these terms and their meanings to persons with disabilities. This could be a reciprocal process with persons with disabilities assisting disability researchers to understand about the context and language used by the context to address persons with disabilities while disability researchers assist persons with disabilities with research skills.

10.3.5 Packaging of Research Findings

Disability researchers and practitioners are requesting improved method of packaging and dissemination of research findings, and this should be in a way that policymakers can easily use. Each context needs to be analysed about the best suitable method that will quickly draw up the attention of the intended audience. Some researchers suggested policy briefs coupled with direct engagement with stakeholders.

10.3.6 Exploration of Neglected Areas in Disability Research

Disability researchers and practitioners were also concerned about neglected areas in disability research. Predictors for stunted growth because of under-nutrition amongst children were of concern which could create a challenge in not delineating whether severity of disability was exacerbated by poor nutrition. The area of assistive technology especially its legislation within the region raised concern. There is a general neglect of research focused on communication and assistive technology to assist communication. There is scarcity of research for persons with disabilities and when this is available it lacks sensitivity towards disability. There are also Maternal health services and data that are not practical disability sensitive, and the language used is usually derogatory. There are also neglected causes of disability (e.g. river blindness), when this is not followed regarding its cause, it is a challenge to obtain methods of intervention.

10.3.7 Development of Disability Research Centres of Excellency

Disability researchers and practitioners were advocating for disability centres of excellence to be developed in different regions. Some were sharing the joys and satisfactions of establishing such units in their areas. This research unit was linked with an association of disabled person's organizations. There was a call upon Governments both in the North and in Africa to support the development of Centres of Excellence that will facilitate the creativity of persons with disabilities, and manage, disseminate and utilize research results. It is encouraged that such units should facilitate private–public sector partnerships on programmes of benefit to and/or led by persons with disabilities in Africa.

10.4 Discussion

Researchers advocated for the use of different methods that could improve rigor in disability research. They recognized the value of both qualitative methods with small sample size that could afford in-depth exploration and description of the lived experiences of persons with disabilities and provide explanations which helps in the building African disability theories. While quantitative methods were seen as providing the much-needed statistics, Kaycee et al. (2022) acknowledge the contribution of big data sets in disability research but warn of substantial limitations that can impede the internal and external validity of a study and some of these limitations include inconsistencies of the definition of disability. While in qualitative research, researchers need to ensure that aspects that are related to accessibility are addressed in the planning for the research (Watharow & Wayland, 2021).

It appears that participatory emancipatory research methodologies are seen as approaches that could bring positive outcomes in disability research. This thinking is supported by Kitchin (2005) who explains that that both participatory (seeking 'positive' individual change through participation) and emancipatory (seeking 'positive' societal change) are empowering. This view jars strongly with that of traditional disability researchers who frequently ignores imbalance of power within the research process and the privileged position of the researcher to set the agenda and control the project outcomes. There are challenges with participatory research methodologies and researchers need to come prepared to have the project agenda rightfully shift according to the needs of participants and the community. Sometimes it might be necessary to expand budget and time to develop research products, or undertake side projects, which are identified by community members as being of prime importance (even when they are secondary to the main research objective) (Gray et al., 2001). Lenette (2022) points to challenges of depth as the researcher must cater for different needs and sometimes larger numbers.

Decolonizing disability research from the region appears to be a commitment from disability researchers. They want to undertake research and plans based on their own African theories, with understanding, and promotion of indigenous knowledge systems as a source of information. This is congruent with Ned et al. (2022) thinking of the need to reimagined disability study and part of this is about the centring of African experiences, voices and knowledges. This is especially so as there are African concepts that are not rigorously pursued in research. Grech (2015) asserts that 'debates and alliances' are vital to the decolonial project and that within transnational collaborations (including between Global South and Global North): [W]e may paradoxically start to challenge the colonial discourse of othering and difference. The decolonial process must also be accepted as messy and continuous and must hold at its centre the recognition of histories of decolonial resistance in particular contexts. They encouraged to enter and play a role in critical discursive inquiry and made a case for understanding the construction of disability discourse and rhetoric in efforts to dismantle disablist constructs (Botha & Ohajunwa, 2024).

Able-bodied disability researchers are encouraged to support disabled people in research skills. There was a perception from disability researchers and practitioners that the key ingredient in advancing the inclusion of persons with disabilities was research skills development, addressing the role of power dynamics, structural and systemic ableism. Botha, Fischer-Mogensen and Brand (2023) point to the need to recognize social exclusion as a much more dynamic problem, and that effectively addressing it is likely not to be achievable within one programme across a single project cycle, but would require a much larger, concerted effort from systemic partners. Attempts in the past were made by late Phiri (2014) with support from Swartz (2014) to initiate a training research program for persons with disabilities. Such programs are rarely sustained as most of the time they depend on external funding.

There were concerns regarding dissemination of research findings and researchers were requesting improved method of packaging, and this should be in a way that policymakers can easily use. This is an important concern that require some innovative ideas. There are seven AfriNEAD conferences that have been hosted except for the publication in special issues, articles in journals and chapters in books what else should AfriNEAD has done to advance this area? The development of AfriNEAD DRCWGs in various countries affiliated to AfriNEAD might be a solution to address this critical area. The DRCWGs could ensure that after AfriNEAD conference participants, take the resolutions to their countries and hold a round table discussion with government to ensure that the resolutions are influencing disability policies in their countries. AfriNEAD conference attendees keep repeating the same items in AfriNEAD research and resolutions in each conference.

There is also a perception from these researchers and practitioners that there are some areas that are neglected in disability research. For example, one hardly see research on predictors for stunted growth because of under-nutrition amongst children were a concern; this could create a challenge in not delineating whether severity of disability has been exacerbated by poor nutrition. It is an already known fact of the struggles of families that encase persons with disabilities and how these families run from pillar to post trying to secure resources that could support their families (Duma et al., 2023). This leaves these families with minimal quality time they could spend with their disabled child.

Finally, these disability researchers are advocating for development of disability research centres of excellence for disability research. These Centres of Excellency should ensure that Disabled People Organizations (DPOs) are central in the initial stages of the development process of these centres. One researcher shared the start of this type of Centre in their area and the joy it has brought to persons with disabilities. Such centres could contribute to the development of African theories on disability that are urgently needed. Grech (2015) affirms that such theories will provide the landscape for understanding contemporary southern spaces within which disability is constructed and lived. Much as there had been questioning in this chapter on disability theories that are emerging from the West and North, a warning has been given of throwing the baby with the bath water. Grech (2015) further asserts that 'debates and alliances' are vital to the decolonial project and that within transnational collaborations (including between Global South and Global North): [W]e may paradoxically start to challenge the colonial discourse of Othering and difference. The decolonial process with its history of resistance could be about persons with disabilities and their families finding their voices in the development of a tapestry for future disability studies in the region.

10.5 Chapter Conclusion

There is a need to recognize that the area of disability research always raises some important and perhaps uncomfortable questions. Partnerships and collaborations have been suggested as a way of levelling out the play-field between persons with disabilities and the abled body people. It is important to enter these difficult conversations to address some of the hidden approaches of power dynamics.

The conference resolutions offer some aspects to consider. What is clear is that there is a need for change in relationships between researchers from different continents and the region this might include using methodologies that can assist in bringing sustainability to the research agenda in the region. Sustainability will assist in building communities of trust in disability research with balance in power and more sustained production of information which could assist in understanding the African story of disability.

A complex picture has emerged from disability researchers that need putting in place some change processes. Central to addressing these complex issues is the need to focus on systems that keep persons with disabilities unable to enjoy their full rights to participate and be part of a transforming African terrain whether it is in rural, urban or peri-urban area.

References

Botha, M., Fischer-Mogensen, K., & Brand, D. (2023). In search of a landing place for persons with disabilities: A critique of South Africa's skills development programme. *The International Journal of Discrimination and the Law, 23*(1–2). https://doi.org/10.1177/13582291231162315

Botha, M., & Ohajunwa, C. (2024). Seeing the human behind the research: Strengthening emerging African disability researchers. *African Journal of Disability, 13*, Article a1494. https://doi.org/10.4102/ajod.v13i0.1494

Dwadwa-Henda, N. (2023). *"Experiences of persons with disabilities of Xhosa rituals and traditions, which contribute to health and wellbeing", PhD thesis* (Issue March) [Open Access, Stellenbosch University]. https://scholar.sun.ac.za/handle/10019.1/128429

Duma, V., Tshabalala, N., & Mji, G. (2021). The black hole of dealing with a disability diagnosis: Views of South African rural parents. *AJOD, 10*, 951. https://doi.org/10.4102/ajod.v10i0.951

Gray, R. E., Fitch, M., Davis C., & Phillips, C. (2001, 25 December). Challenges of participatory research: Reflections on a study with breast cancer self-help groups. *Health Expect, 3*(4), 243–252. https://doi.org/10.1046/j.1369-6513.2000.00100.x

Grech, S. (2015). Decolonising Eurocentric disability studies: Why colonialism matters in the disability and Global South debate. *Social Identities, 21*(1), 6–21. https:// doi.org/https://doi.org/10.1080/13504630.2014.995347

Kaycee, B. L., & Mills, B. (2022). Limitations when conducting quantitative disability research. *Journal of Research Initiatives, 6*(2), Article 10. Retrieved from https://digitalcommons.uncfsu.edu/jri/vol6/iss2/10

Kachaje, R., Dube, K., MacLachlan, M., & Mji, G. (2014). The African network for evidence-to-action on disability: A role player in the realisation of the UNCRPD in Africa. *AJOD, 3*(2).

Kitchin, R. (2005). *Towards emancipatory and empowering disability research: reflections on three participatory action research projects*. National University of Ireland Maynooth.

Lenette, C. (2022). What does participation entail? Challenges to genuine participation in participatory action research. In Lenette, chapter 7 pg. 41–59. Oxford University Press Oxford. doi.org/https://doi.org/10.1093/oso/978 0197512456.003.0003

Masaka, D. (2018). *The Prospects of Ending Epistemicide in Africa: Some Thoughts Journal of Black Studies, 49*(3), 284–301.

Mji, G., & Edusei, A. (2019). *An Introduction to a Special Issue on the Role of Assistive Technology in Social Inclusion of Persons with Disabilities in Africa: Outcome of the Fifth African Network for Evidence-to-Action in Disability Conference Afr J Disabil*. https://doi.org/10.4102/ajod.v8i0.681

Mji, G., MacLachlan, M., Melling-Williams, N., & Gcaza, S. (2009). Realising the rights of disabled people in Africa: An introduction to the special issue. *Disability and Rehabilitation Journal.*

Mji, G., & Ohajunwa, C. (2021). *Ubuntu ethics and human rights: Implications for rehabilitation practices in indigenous African families of persons with disabilities (PWDs)*. Midrand KR Publishing.

Ned, L. Y., Dube, K., & Swartz, L. (2022). Challenges and opportunities of centring the African voice in disability research. *African Journal of Disability, 11*, Article a1089. https://doi.org/10.4102/ajod.v11i0.1089

Ohajunwa, C. O., Mji, G., & Chimbala-Kalenga, R. (2022). Encouraging reciprocal healthcare practice within a South African Indigenous community. *AlterNative: An International Journal of Indigenous Peoples, 18*(1), 141–146. https://doi.org/10.1177/11771801221085631

Ohajunwa, C. O., & Sefotho, M. M. (2024). Epistemologies of disability from the Global South: Towards good health. In The Routledge International Handbook of Disability and Global Health. Lieketseng Ned, Minerva Rivas Verlade, Satendra Singh, Leslie Swartz and Karen Soldatic (Eds). ISBN 9781032131849. 10,4324/9781003228059

Phiri, A. M. (2014). Building communities of trust: Challenges for disability. *African Journal of Disability, 3*(2), Art. #77, 3. https://doi.org/10.4102/ajod.v3i2.77

Sefotho, M. M. (2021). Basotho ontology of disability: An afrocentric onto-epistemology. *Heliyon, 7*(3), 8. https://doi.org/10.1016/j.heliyon.2021.e06540

South African White Paper on Integrated National Disability Strategy. (1997). Republic of South Africa.

Swartz, L. (2014). Five challenges for disability-related research in sub-Saharan Africa. *African Journal of Disability, 3*(2), 149.

Watharow, A., & Wayland, S. (2001). Making qualitative research inclusive: methodological insights in disability research. *Health Expectations, 3*(4), 243–252. https://doi.org/10.1046/j.1369-6513.2000.00100.x

Appendix 1: Guideline for Researchers and Research Ethics Committees (RECs)

GUIDELINE FOR RESEARCHERS AND RESEARCH ETHICS COMMITTEES (RECs)
The taking, storage, distribution and publication of photographs in vulnerable populations
Developed by Gubela Mji and Nicola Bardorf (2013)

Researchers proposing to use photographs in their research must commit to:

1. Use photographs as a research tool/aid only if the photo(s) will contribute something positive, significant, meaningful and/or substantive to the research question; or that the photo(s) may, through highlighting visually, offer benefit to or promote the rights of a particular group.
2. Respect research participants in the handling of the photograph(s).
3. Develop and implement a standardized protocol, included as part of the submission to the Research Ethics Committee, for the use of photographs during fieldwork.
4. Develop and implement procedures to maintain the confidentiality of information collected, including the safe storage of all research photographs in a regulated environment with controlled access.

G. Mji (ed.), *Doing Disability Research in Africa*,
https://doi.org/10.1007/978-3-031-98549-2

5. Devote time and resources to awareness-raising in the research team of how to ethically manage photos.
6. Obtain fully informed consent (IC) to take and use photographs in the research before the photo(s) are taken. While it would be preferable to get informed consent before, in cases where this may alter the 'real' nature of the photo, minimally consent after the photo is taken and before the photo is used is necessary.
7. Explain during informed consent discussions and in the informed consent document:

   - The standardized protocol for the use of photographs during fieldwork.
   - the need for and contribution the photo(s) will make to the study.
   - how the photo(s) will be used e.g. report writing, presentations, conferences, meetings, journal publications, social media.
   - any anticipated wider implications of their publication.
   - any anticipated consequences for participants.
   - how the photo(s) will be securely stored to protect confidentiality.
   - that the participant can receive a copy of the photo; and
   - that the participant can withdraw the photo at any time.

8. Protect participant privacy through:

   - anonymization or de-identification of photographs, where appropriate. Complete anonymity is not always possible and the minimum area of the body, or minimal identifiable features necessary will be captured; and
   - avoiding signs, or other readily identifiable objects, in the immediate environment, in photos that might deny individuals anonymity and inadvertently allow others to locate them in the community.

9. Obtain informed consent for each intended use of the photo prior to publication:

   - allow the participant to review the photo(s) and any accompanying text descriptions or draft articles before the photos are published; and

- allow confirmation from the participant of whether the photo is an accurate/appropriate representation, considered culturally acceptable, and will likely not lead to further stigma or discrimination prior to publication.

Index

G. Mji (ed.), *Doing Disability Research in Africa*,
https://doi.org/10.1007/978-3-031-98549-2

Kolibri 360 GmbH
Ferdinand-Jühlke-Straße 7
99095 Erfurt, Deutschland
produktsicherheit@kolibri360.de